The Diet of Eden

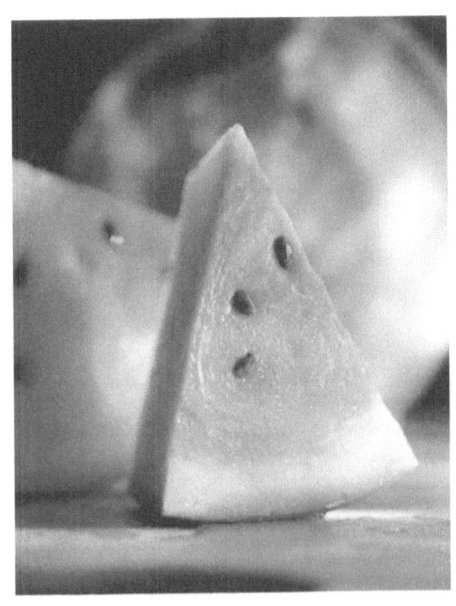

The Diet of Eden

How the Low-Carbohydrate Diets Almost Had It Right

Pam Warmerdam, MS, RD, CDE

To order additional copies of this book, contact:
Xlibris Corporation
1-888-795-4274
www.Xlibris.com
Orders@Xlibris.com

or go to www.nutritionstudio.net
or call toll free at 1-877-598-1589

About the Author

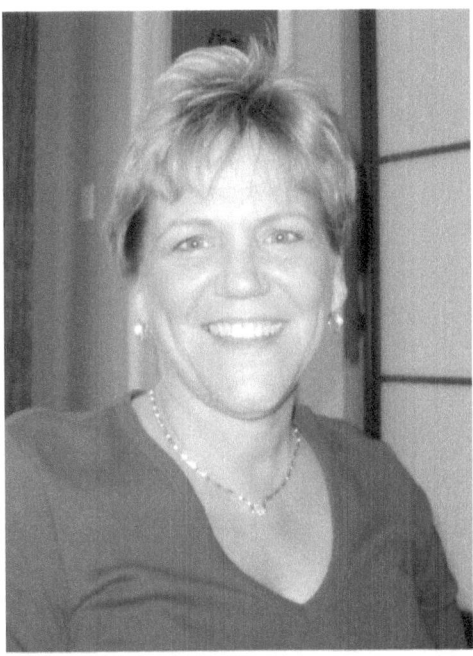

Born and raised in a small town in central Ohio, Pam watched her family struggle intensively with weight, diabetes, heart disease, and strokes.

The first in her immediate family to attend college, it was with her first class in nutrition that she decided this was to be her career.

Throughout her college and career, she has specialized in weight control and diabetes education. She has a bachelors and a master of science (MS) degree in nutrition and has been a registered dietician (RD) since 1987. She has worked in managerial positions in different hospitals, but has always managed to find time to work in the field of weight loss counseling that she loved so well. She has been a certified diabetes educator (CDE) since 1999.

In 2002, she opened her own business, the Nutrition Studio & Diabetes Care Center, and has helped thousands of people to learn to eat a healthier, more natural diet.

In 2010, Pam decided to change the type of business from sole ownership to a non-profit corporation. This decision was a difficult one, as she had put years of hard work into the business and as a non-profit organization, she no longer had ownership of it.

However, this is something she felt she had to do because she was unable to get insurance companies to contract with her to provide these services and was having to turn away between 40 - 50% of the diabetic patients that were being referred to her. She is hoping that by opening the business as a non-profit, she will be able to obtain grants from various sources and will no longer have to turn those patients away who need nutrition and diabetes education.

Acknowledgments

First of all, I would like to thank my best female friend, Janice, for her undying support and encouragement during the writing of this book. I was tempted to give up several times, but she would have no part of it.

I would also like to thank my daughter, Alison, who fearlessly endured the trial recipes; not all of which were successes.

Additional thanks go to my assistant, Rebecca, who never stops amazing me with her initiative and support and to Lauren, a nutrition student who helped with the research for the book. Finally I would like to thank my family in Ohio and all of my patients in California, whose own struggles with weight and/or diabetes continue to inspire me to want to help.

Preface

Or do you not know that your body is a temple of the
holy spirit within you, whom you have from God?

1 Corinthians 6:19 ESV

For My Mom

The Early Days:

One of my mother's earliest childhood memories was being shoved
from her father's lap at the age of three, being told she was getting "too
big" for him. In her young mind, she truly believed he didn't love her
because she was too fat.

Born the last of five children and the only girl, she was my
grandmother's final hope at connecting with this emotionally distant
man. Yet as the Bible says in Exodus 20:5, the way a man lives his life will
somehow affect the next several generations of his family thereafter.

My grandfather's inability to show his love to this sensitive and
bright little girl set the stage for a life filled with a struggle to be thin, a
struggle to feel accepted, a struggle to be loved. Her mother sensed this
in her young daughter and tried to make her feel better the only way
she knew how—by making special treats and buying her clothes.

My mom was born into a family with both parents being
overweight (her father both overweight and a type 2 diabetic). She
too had her share of baby fat. Her round, chubby cheeks and pudgy
arms and legs gave her four older brothers plenty of ammunition for
the teasing and taunting that siblings are apt to do.

High School:

It was the summer between Mom's junior and senior year that she
discovered that by swimming for four hours per day and eating only
one small meal in the evening, she was finally able to lose weight. She
became a slender and beautiful young woman with measurements of
38-24-42. She had developed into a very bright and ambitious woman,
who was going to graduate from high school with top honors, and had
already bought herself a car with money she had made and saved over
the years through babysitting, tutoring, etc. She had dreams of going to
medical school.

It was during her senior year at a basketball game that she saw the man with whom she would spend the rest of her life. He was tall, slender, and dashingly handsome. He was sitting on the bench with a broken arm. She nudged her best friend, smiled at him across the room, and said, "I'm going to marry that guy." Sure enough, a little over a year later, she was pregnant and they were married.

It was too early for this handsome young man to get tied down, but he wanted to do the right thing. No matter where he went, girls were attracted to him like vultures to a carcass.

She gained quite a bit during that first pregnancy. She went from working and swimming every day to being a housewife. Her husband would often be out drinking with his friends, so she was lonely. When the baby was born, her mom came to take care of her, the only way she knew how.

To add to this, her new mother-in-law, a status-seeking socialite, already had planned out the life of her son, an only child. She had already chosen another woman to be his wife and had arranged many dates between them, going as far as buying them matching shirts for when they went out. She was devastated by this unplanned pregnancy and marriage and never failed to show her distain to this girl who had dashed her dreams for her beautiful son.

Four Years Later, Age Twenty-Two:

Now with two children and pregnant again, she discovered her husband was having an affair with the babysitter, who was about the same age as this young couple. By this time, she had gained about forty pounds. She figured her weight was again the reason this man did not love her. She started smoking. In her depression, she even considered aborting this third child (if she had, you wouldn't be reading this). She might have divorced him, but her mom told her she had "made her own bed" and needed to live with the consequences.

Age Forty-Two:

Yes! A new diet, martinis and whipped cream, promised you could eat all the fattening stuff you liked to eat—like bacon, butter, and juicy steaks—and still lose weight. By then, she had tried all kinds of diet crazes, from the Scarsdale diet to a chocolate candy called Ayds. She had lost and regained hundreds of pounds. She was also smoking two packs of cigarettes per day. It was then she had her first heart attack.

It was relatively silent, just persistent pain in her neck and chest and an overall feeling of tiredness and not feeling well. She figured if she went to the doctor, he would just tell her it was her nerves and that she should lose weight. Her doctor actually found the heart attack about a year later on an electrocardiogram.

Age Forty-Five:
Her twenty-year-old daughter was interviewing her for a college class about aging. She revealed to her daughter that she truly believed she would not live past fifty (her father had a massive fatal heart attack when he was fifty-four). At this point, she was through with dieting and was just going to enjoy eating whatever she wanted.

Age Sixty-Two:
She was hospitalized yet again for congestive heart failure. Her HMO sent her home without saying anything about diabetes. Her blood sugar was 362.

Age Sixty-Six:
She could tell it was another heart attack. She called her husband from work to take her to the hospital, then panicked and called 911. They rushed her to the hospital and determined that it was a heart attack and gave her an emergency angiogram. Although she had allergic reactions to the dyes injected during the procedure in the past, the doctors felt it needed to be done to save her life. She reacted negatively to the dye and her kidneys shut down. Her heart could not handle the fluids, and she again went into congestive heart failure and this time was placed on a ventilator. Her family was called in from around the country as she was not expected to live. She had tubes and bags hanging everywhere. She then suffered a stroke on top of all of this, yet manages to pull through.

Age Sixty-Nine:
Mom had a rough year. Although she had made it through the rehab hospitals and was back in her home, she was now on a multitude of medicines including insulin. She stood up only to get to her power scooter and back to bed. She had neuropathy in her feet and would often scream out in pain.

On Thanksgiving, she cried at her daughter's house when she was unable to stand up after going to the toilet and had to get help from her son-in-law.

Her daughter visited from California. The house was dirty and smelled of urine. Mom was sitting at the table in her power scooter, drinking a (regular) Pepsi, and smoking a cigarette while wearing her oxygen mask. She had truly given up. It was hard to watch. Her daughter, who had become a dietitian and had studied weight loss and diabetes for twenty-five years, was at a loss. She thought about a line from the movie *Cool Hand Luke*: "Some folks you just can't reach."

Later in that same trip, her daughter sat in her mom's bedroom and tried to share with her some new theories about weight and diabetes. Her mom usually devours this type of discussion, but she barely listens. Her skin was gray and pasty. Her other three daughters were coming over for lunch that day. She came out to the kitchen in her scooter and ate her lunch but got more and more tired. She became short of breath and started to panic, so we again called an ambulance.

She never made it out of the hospital this time. She died a slow and agonizing death. Her daughter vowed to get the word out about this disease that predominated in the life of this woman.

Note:

There were two things that happened around the time of my mother's demise that made it easier to deal with much of the tragedy of her life and death.

The first happened around six months prior to Mom's death. It happened during the relaxation portion of my yoga class. We were lying prone on our yoga mats, with the lights low and soft, relaxing music playing in the background.

Our instructor was leading us through a visualization exercise. While we were in this relaxed state, she had us picture someone's eyes (the window to their soul she describes). Immediately my mom's eyes came to mind. The instructor had us picture the color (pale sky blue), the shape, and the skin around the eyes. She then told us to look deeper into those eyes and try to see what those eyes are saying about the person.

What I saw in my mother's eyes was sadness. It was a sadness of someone who seemed to have lived her life never feeling truly loved. When I sat up from the relaxation period, tears were streaming down my face. There were several others in the class who were also crying, so I felt in good company.

I went home that day and got on the computer to send my mom an instant message (IM). This was her favorite mode of communication at the time. I described my experience to her, but added that there was someone who loved her unconditionally, fully, and without hesitation. Of course, I meant God. She reassured me that she knew this, and I felt more at peace for her.

The second thing happened around three years after my mom's death. She came back to me in one of my dreams. She was absolutely beautiful. She was young, thin, healthy, and energetic. She told me she was walking every day. I asked her why she didn't do this while she was still here on earth. She simply explained to me, "Because now I have no pain." Even in her death, she was helping me to learn and understand my own clients better.

Contents

Chapter 1

Introduction

As medical professionals, we used to think excess weight caused diabetes, high blood pressure, and high cholesterol. While there may be a relationship between being overweight and these diseases, many researchers and medical experts now believe that many people are born with an inborn susceptibility to gain weight easily. I call this a genetic predisposition for overweight (GPO). This condition has been called insulin resistance, metabolic syndrome, or syndrome X. For simplicity's sake, I will refer to it as GPO, and I will explain more about the syndrome in upcoming pages.

It is estimated that as many as 25 to 50 percent of the American population is predisposed to this condition. If you are of certain ethnic backgrounds, such as Hispanic, African American, Asian, or American Indian, the incidence is even higher. Perhaps it is that the closer our ancestors were to living off the land, the less likely we are to tolerate mankind's processed foods.

When you see an overweight child, there is a good chance he or she has GPO. This is not to ignore the other causes of excess weight such as stressful lifestyles; too little activity; too much time with TVs, video games, or computers; and too many processed foods. But these things alone cannot explain why two children can eat similar foods, get similar activity, and one might weigh significantly more than the other.

God provides for us all we need on earth to survive. The more we alter our environment (including our foods), the more we tend to offset the balance of God's intended nature. With the natural balance so off-kilter, we are going to see our health become worse and worse.

And God said, *"See, I have given you every herb that yields seed which is on the face of the earth, and every tree whose fruit yields seed; to you it shall be for food"* (Genesis 1:29).

What Is The Diet of Eden?

The Diet of Eden may just become the new hip and trendy plan, possibly because of its simplicity, and because it works. It is based on a plan that was originally devised a long, long time ago—looking at what God put here on earth for us to survive and thrive.

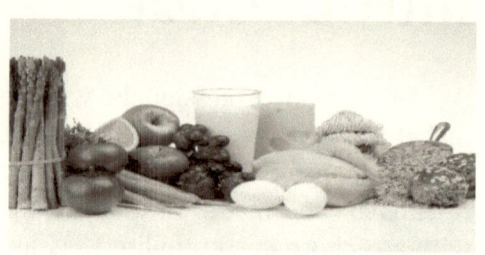

The The Diet of Eden is a diet of abundance. Picture in your mind a feast of foods that were put on earth by God—a diet full of nuts, whole grains, beautiful and colorful fruits, and vegetables. Our bodies are meant to consume foods supplied by nature.

Now picture a diet of foods eaten by many typical Americans:

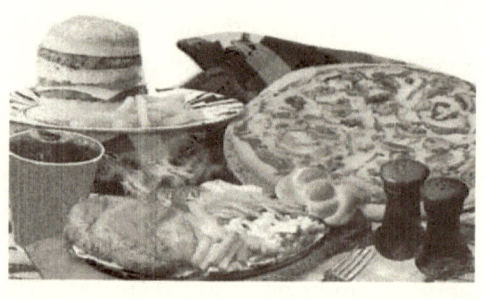

Just how many of these foods are recognizable from nature? There are a couple of tomatoes and a few patches of green, but for the most part, these foods bear little resemblance to their natural forms.

As a registered dietitian (RD) with a passion for helping others lose weight, I am painfully aware of all of the different types of diets available on the market

- Very low-calorie liquid diets
- Low fat
- High protein, low carbohydrate
- Protein sparing

- Over-the-counter or physician-prescribed appetite suppressants
- Calorie or fat-gram counting
- Exchange system (diabetic diet)
- Weight-loss surgery

Although other diets may come and go throughout the years, almost all plans are a variation of one of the above diets.

Like fashion, most diets tend to run their twenty-year cycles. For example, the low-carbohydrate diet was popularized in the 1970s with the martinis and whipped cream plan and made its comeback in the 1990s to early 2000s with the "new and improved" Atkins plan.

The dieting industry is a multibillion dollar business, yet touts overall only a 5 percent long-term success rate. If only everyone would adopt the motto of our own organization:

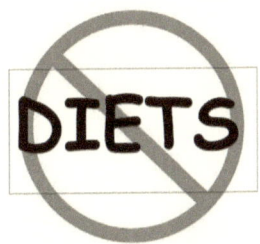

**If it's not a PLAN
You think you CAN (stick with)
JUST DON'T DO IT!**

The high-protein, low-carbohydrate diets, such as the Atkins diet were likely some of the most highly controversial diet plans ever proposed. With claims to be able to eat all of the meat, cheese, butter, and cream, and still lose weight, they certainly sounded like a plan many people could follow. And many certainly did.

Thousands, if not millions, of people devoured these diets with gusto. Many people experienced weight loss results almost immediately, losing several pounds within the first week.

The problem is that these diets were pretty much in direct conflict with what most of the medical community was prescribing for a healthy diet. Research was becoming clearer to indicate the correlation between certain types of fats and high cholesterol levels and heart disease. On top of this, fats carry almost twice the number of calories as the other nutrients, so a low-fat, high-carbohydrate diet was being recommended by the majority of medical professionals, with fats ranging from between 10 to 30 percent of the total calories.

Could these low-carbohydrate diets indeed cause people to lose weight? Were they indeed as safe and effective as their creators suggested? Obviously, the answer to the first question was yes. People were seeing their friends and coworkers lose weight with a plan that was clearly spelled out, relatively easy to follow, and pretty tasty. But was the diet safe? This is a question that is still a highly controversial one.

Personally, I also like to look at diets from a more philosophical stance. Does the plan make sense in view of our lives as God (or nature, if you prefer) intended?

Create in me a clean heart, oh Lord;
And renew a right spirit within me.

—Psalm 51:10

Chapter 2

How the Low Carbohydrate Diets Almost Had It Right

Confusion about Diets

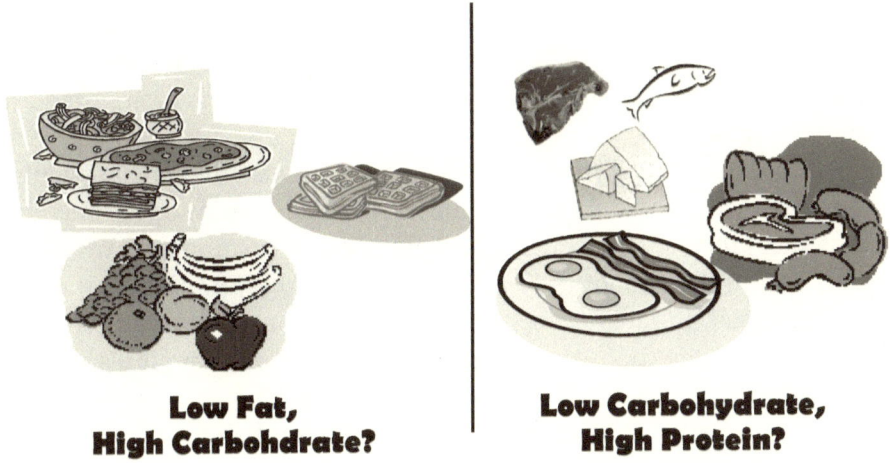

Low Fat, High Carbohdrate?

Low Carbohydrate, High Protein?

Every diet that has been introduced over the years probably has some redeeming qualities. As far as the low carbohydrate diets are concerned, any diet that can get people from drinking regular sodas and eating mass-produced pastries cannot be all bad.

Most people who tried the low carbohydrate diets experienced successful weight loss if they were able to follow them. Those with this genetic predisposition for overweight (GPO) likely experienced the most success with these diets.

One of the main problems with the low carbohydrate diets is that calories come from three (3) main nutrients: carbohydrates, proteins and fats. If the carbohydrates are significantly restricted, this leaves proteins and fats.

In some of the original low carbohydrate diets, there were unlimited amounts of high saturated fats, such as bacon, sausage, heavy creams, etc. These saturated fats, eaten in excess, are found to raise cholesterol levels and lead to clogging of the arteries.

Therefore, in the "new and improved" versions of the low carbohydrate diets, mostly lean meats were recommended, such as chicken, fish and lean cuts of beef. Although this seemed to be an improvement, it left most of the calories being consumed coming from pure protein.

Unfortunately, this is a problem because if protein is eaten in excess, the kidneys can be negatively affected, as there is a threshold to the amount of protein the kidneys can handle.

Another reason these low carb diets produced results is due to the lack of availability of high protein, low carbohdrate foods. After all, when was the last time you went to a meeting and was offered a plateful of chicken?

More than likely, when attending meetings or other social events, foods that are offered would be muffins, bagels, sandwiches and the like. Unless the dieter planned ahead far enough to bring their own low carb, high protein food, they would likely do without that particular meal or snack. In fact, it has been found that the average intake on a low carbohydrate diet was around 1200 calories, making it also a low calorie diet.

But my reason for questioning the rationale behind the low carb diets goes beyond the science. It is also a question of following the natural order of God's intentions for us. God put on earth all that we really need to survive and thrive. God made fruits and vegetables, so it seems wrong to think we should not eat them.

God made a potato (but did not make potato chips and french fries). God made whole grains and brown rice. Many people are surprised to find out that white rice has been processed by man. I believe that whenever we eat white rice, white flour or white noodles, it reacts similarly to eating pure white sugar.

Don't get me wrong, I believe I understand why man learned to process our foods. It helped them to remain shelf-stable for a longer period of time.

Inside a whole grain, whether wheat, rice, or corn, there is something called the germ. This is not like a bacteria-type of germ, but it is the part of the grain that contains some very healthy oils, such as the omega 3 oils.

Unfortunately, however, oils are not shelf stable and will turn rancid over time, so man learned that if he was to first remove the bran layer of the grain, he could get to and remove the germ. This leaves only the endosperm which is primarily carbohydrates and a small amount of protein. (See chapter 7 you can find a chart which outlines the difference in nutrients between a whole grain and one that has been processed.)

So now, with the germ removed, the grain is quite shelf stable. This was actually quite a good deal for people in third world countries. We were now able to send grains such as rice to these countries and feed multitudes of starving people.

Unfortunately, the people who were fed these processed grains were still falling ill and dying of malnutrition, due to the lack of nutrients which had been removed in the processing. That is why these processed grains became "enriched". This term simply means that some of the nutrients which were removed in the processing were added back.

Now people in starving countries could be kept alive on these processed grains.

The problems arose when these processed grains were introduced into countries who had no food shortages. These grains provide plenty of calories, but less nutrients in a form that is easily stored by the body.

Although the high protein, low carbohydrate diets did get people away from these processed carbohydrates, they also took away the natural carbohydrates that God put on earth for energy and enjoyment, such as our fruits, vegetables, and whole grains. In addition to that, the high protein, low carbohydrate diets can, over time, provide an overload of protein which can adversely affect our kidneys. God provided us with all we need for our bodies to flourish, and meant for us to eat these foods in balance.

> Every moving thing that lives shall be food for you. As I gave you the green plants, I give you everything. -Genesis 9:3

Chapter 3

Causes of Overweight in Modern times

In this chapter I will discuss the multi-faceted array of reasons to help explain why we are seeing more obesity than ever.

Most of you are likely aware of the alarming rise in the rate of obesity in our country. To view this in an astonishing format, try the typing the following site into your computer search engine: mpkb.org/_detail/home/pathogenesis/obesity-1985-2009-cdc.gif

Causes of Overweight in Modern Times

1. Genetic predisposition to overweight (GPO)

This will be decribed in greater detail in chapter 6.

2. Stressful lifestyles

Many families consist of a single parent or of both parents who need to work to make ends meet. Stress has become a part of our everyday lives. Stress alone can make the body over-produce insulin by stimulating our stress hormones (cortisol and norepinephrine). Over-production of insulin can cause weight gain.

With both parents working full-time jobs and commuting long hours, there is less time available for planning and preparing healthy meals. If the kids are in multiple sports, this can take even more time away from family meals.

When I was a child, dining out was a special occasion. We were lucky to go out more than once every six months!

Today, it is rare to find a family who goes out to eat less than once a week. In fact, I have seen families who eat fifteen out of twenty-one meals per week away from home. (I consider most school lunches and cafeteria eating to be dining out.) Along with stressful lifestyles, larger portions and more dining out can have a cumulative negative effect on our overall health.

Not only are families likely overeating calories and suboptimal amount of nutrients from restaurant foods, we are less likely to be teaching our children how to cook. I cannot tell you how many twenty-somethings who have come to my office looking for nutrition advice that have culinary skills for little more than boxed macaroni and cheese and ramen noodles.

We need to take the time to make and enjoy healthier meals and snacks. Rather than counting calories and restricting ourselves on the amount of processed foods we eat, wouldn't it be better to eat a diet of abundance which our Father has provided? It is <u>what</u> we eat that will make a huge difference.

> Better is a dinner of herbs where love is than a fattened ox and hatred with it.
>
> -Proverbs 15:17

3. Less activity

I often hear people say, "My great-grandparents ate eggs, bacon, biscuits and gravy for breakfast almost every morning and they were not overweight". But these same grandparents were likely much more active than we are. Our ancestors often had to work the land and even pump and carry their own water.

As kids, we were much more likely to be able to run around with our friends than kids are able to these days. Founded or not, parents tend to have more fear of allowing their children to play outside than previous generations. Therefore, children tend to spend more time indoors and often in front of a TV, video game or computer.

For the most part, exercise is no longer a natural part of living in our current society; it now needs to be planned and scheduled into our lives.

4. Processed, fast foods and increased portion sizes

The food processing industry spends billions of dollars advertising these man-made and man-altered foods. This makes it difficult for natural foods to remain popular or even desired. For instance, when was the last time you saw a commercial for an apple or broccoli?

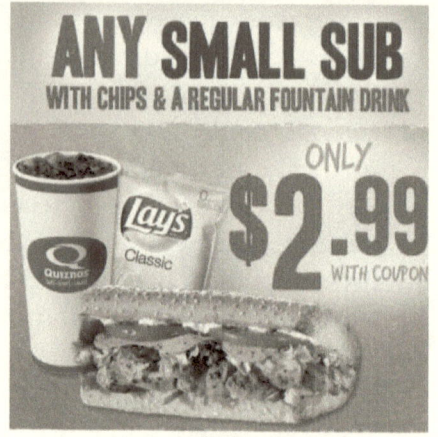

Along with our more stressful lifestyles can come less time to prepare healthful meals. The sheer number of eating establishments in the US has increased by 75% between 1977 & 1991. Processed and fast foods can be cheaper to produce (for instance, they may have a longer shelf life or be "mass" produced).

Typical Fast-Food Meal

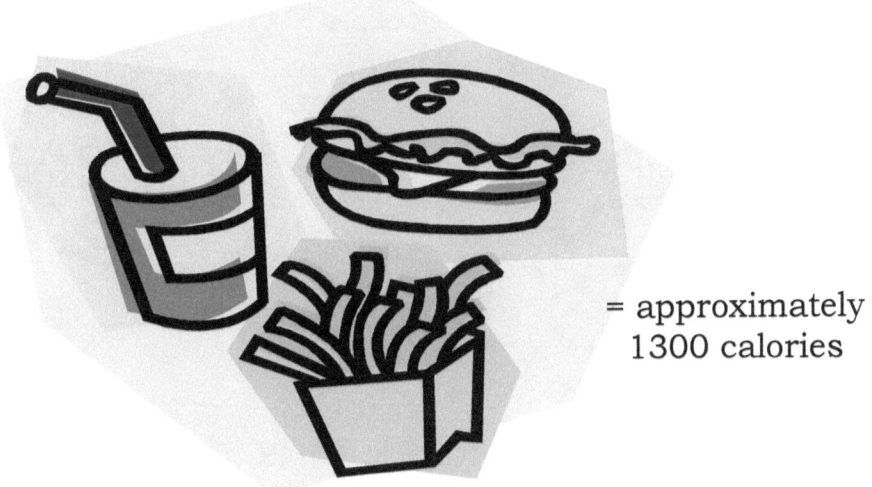

= approximately
1300 calories

For the same calories, you could have had

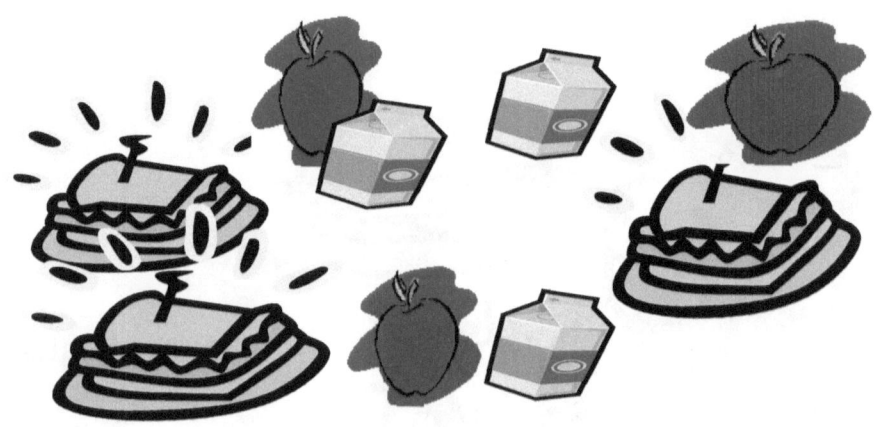

three turkey sandwiches, three apples, and three glasses of milk!

Meal Advertised at a Local Mini-Mart

¼ lb. hotdog

$2.99

Biggie Chips

44 oz. soda

Another name for this meal:

"Where else but America can you get an entire day's worth of calories, sugar and saturated fat for just $2.99?"

• Increased portion sizes

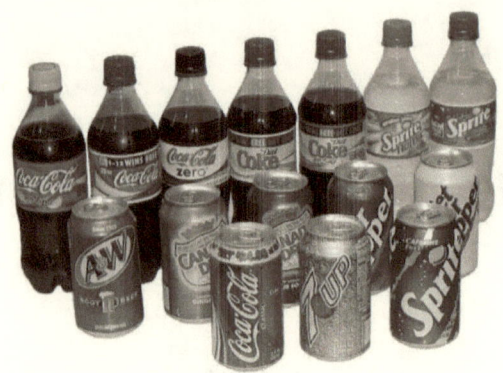

Portion sizes have consistantly gotten larger over the years. Bags of snack foods or soft drinks in vending machines and the grocery store are offered in larger and larger sizes. Most of these items contain multiple servings while a 1-ounce bag of snack food or an 8-ounce soft drink, which are the recommended single serving sizes, are very difficult to find. These larger sizes tend to appeal to our economic sensibilities but also lead to increased calorie intake.

While eating lunch with some nurses whose families originated from the Philippines, I overheard them discussing that when American Filipino children move back to the Philippines, they often need to serve them *two* school lunches. American children have just gotten used to eating a larger quantity of foods, and we're just not doing enough strenuous exercise to be able to burn off these excess calories.

Over the past fifty years, our portions have increased significantly. Back in the 1950s, and even today in certain European countries, a fountain soda consisted of 7 oz. soda and 1 oz. of ice. This comes up to 88 calories. When we order a soda in America, the average serving size is 20 oz. Let's say 3 oz. of this is ice. Therefore this soda now provides 212 calories.

Although you may not think this 124-calorie disparity makes much of a difference, you need to realize that just 100 extra calories per day can add up to a 10-pound weight gain over a year. Therefore this one soda per day can add up to an extra 12.4 pounds of extra weight in a year.

If you add up the differences between a simple hamburger, french fry, and soda meal from the 1950s portions to today's portions, we would find a difference of over 200 calories.

Considering that the average adult female needs approximately 400 to 500 calories per meal, and the average adult male needs approximately 600 to 700 calories per meal (based on the recommended three meals per day and leaving a little for snacks), let's see how a couple of restaurant meals fit into this meal plan.

Restaurant Portion Sizes

Please don't take this wrong; there is nothing terrible about going out to dinner. Getting to choose whatever we want, being waited on, and not having to clean up is an amazing treat. But a treat is how we need to look at dining out, not something we do many times a week. If we are going out more than once a month, we really need to consider dining out like we do our other meals; and take some time and consideration to assure that we are eating healthfully and taking care of our temples (bodies).

Of course, with just a little effort, we could come up with a healthier menu option, even at these same restaurants.

Remember a reduction of 100 calories per day could equal to 10 pounds over a year, so the savings between these two menus could mean as much as 220 pounds.

Good-Day Steakhouse Menu*

½ serving of cheese fries	1,450 calories
porterhouse steak	1,230 calories
sautéed mushrooms	150 calories
fresh vegetable	80 calories
baked potato with butter and cheese	400 calories
½ serving of chocolate dessert	610 calories
large soda or lemonade	478 calories
Total	**4,398 calories**

We are looking at a surplus of about 1,300 to 4,000 excess calories in this one meal! If overeating like this is done on a daily basis, this could potentially add up from 130 to 400 extra pounds in a year.

Good-Day Steakhouse Menu*

side Caesar salad	210 calories
8 oz. filet mignon steak	605 calories
sautéed mushrooms	150 calories
fresh vegetable (double order)	160 calories
large diet soda or water with lemon	0 calories
Total	**1,125 calories**

Although still rather high in calories, this meal saved 3,273 calories.

*Names of restaurants are fictitious; calorie amounts are based on typical restaurants of the sort and are found at CalorieKing.com.

La Mexicana Menu#1*

½ basket chips and salsa	485 calories
2 enchiladas	660 calories
side of beans	160 calories
side of rice	160 calories
sour cream, 2 tbsp.	50 calories
large soda or lemonade (1 refill)	478 calories
Total	**1,993 calories**

La Mexicana Menu#2*

10 chips and salsa (eating slowly)	170 calorie
chicken tostada	360 calories
side of beans	160 calories
sour cream, 2 tbsp.	50 calories
large diet soda or iced tea (1 refill)	0 calories
Total	**740 calories**

Granted, this is still greater than what some of us need in a single meal, but it has significantly fewer calories than the previous menu of this restaurant. We actually avoided eating 1,223 calories over the previous menu.

You may think, "These smaller meals are never going to fill me up", and at first you may be right. You may be accustomed to eating portions that are much larger than needed or recommended.

To help you get used to smaller portions, you might try a trick that one of my patients taught me. I call it the "80% Rule of Eating". You want to eat slowly enough and pay enough attention that you can feel when you are only 80% full (instead of 100% or even 110%).

Then you want to wait 20 minutes. You can even set a timer if you need. Likely you will find that after 20 minutes, your stomach has been able to let your brain know that it has had enough to eat, and you will be perfectly satisfied, but not uncomfortably stuffed.

*Names of restaurants are fictitious; calorie amounts are based on typical restaurants of the sort and are found at CalorieKing.com.

American vs. European Sodas

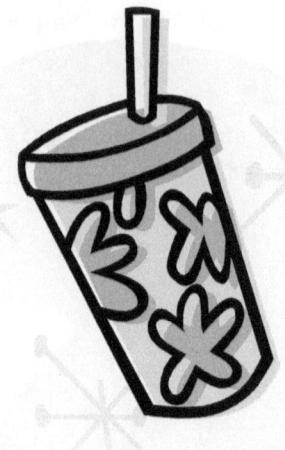

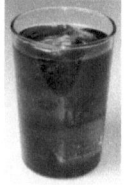

44 oz. = 30 tsp
sugar (480 calories)

8 oz. = 5 ½
tsp. sugar (88 calories)

Remember, it only takes an extra 100 calories per day to cause us to put on an additional 10 pounds of excess weight in a year.

Let's look at how many teaspoons of sugar are contained in many common beverages. You may multiply each teaspoon of sugar by four to come up with the calories from sugar.

How Much Sugar are We Drinking?*

Beverage	Teaspoons of sugar	Grams of Sugar	Calories from sugar
Campbell's V-8 Splash, 12 oz	7 tsp	29 gm	116 sugar calories
Campbell's Diet V-8 Splash, 12 oz	1 tsp	5 gm	20 sugar calories
Campbell's V-8 Vegetable Juice, 12 oz	1 tsp	6 gm	24 sugar calories
Capri Sun, 25% less sugar, 6.75oz	5 tsp	19 gm	76 sugar calories
Capri Sun, 100% Juice, 6.75 oz	6 tsp	24 gm	96 sugar calories
Carrot Juice, 12 oz	5 tsp	20 gm	80 sugar calories
Coca-Cola, 12 oz	10 tsp	39 gm	156 sugar calories
Coca-Cola, Diet, 12 oz	0 tsp	0 gm	0 sugar calories
Cranberry Juice Cocktail, 12 oz	9 tsp	34 gm	136 sugar calories
Cranberry Juice Cocktail, Diet, 12 oz	Less than 1 tsp	3 gm	12 sugar calories
Crystal Light, 12 oz	0 tsp	0 gm	0 sugar calories
Fruit Punch, Sunny D, 12 oz	11 tsp	44 gm	176 sugar calories
Gatorade, 20 oz bottle	8 tsp	32 gm	128 sugar calories
G-2 by Gatorade, 20 oz bottle	4 tsp	17 gm	68 sugar calories
Hi-C Juice Drinks, 12 oz	12 tsp	48 gm	192 sugar calories
Sugar-Free Hawaiian Punch, (added to bottled water) 1 pkt	0 tsp	0 gm	0 sugar calories
Horchata Rice Beverage, 12 oz	9.5 tsp	38 gm	152 sugar calories
Jamba Juice, 24 oz (original size)Classic Smoothie, Banana Berry	22 tsp	86 gm	344 sugar calories
Iced Tea, Sweetened, 12 oz	7 tsp	27 gm	108 sugar calories
Iced Tea, Diet or Unsweetened, 12 oz	0 tsp	2 gm	8 sugar calories

100% Juice (apple, orange, pineapple), 12 oz	11 tsp	45 gm	180 sugar calories
Kern's Nectar, 11.5 oz can	13 tsp	52 gm	208 sugar calories
Kool-Aid, made as directed, 12 oz	6 tsp	24 gm	96 sugar calories
Lemonade, Country Time®, 12 oz prepared	6 tsp	24 gm	96 sugar calories
Propel Fitness Water (by Gatorade), 23 oz bottle	1.5 tsp	48 gm	192 sugar calories
Slurpee or Slushie, Punch or Dr. Pepper flavored, 12 oz	6 tsp	24 gm	96 sugar calories
Slurpee or Slushie, , Punch or Dr. Pepper flavored , 44 oz	40 tsp	160 gm	640 sugar calories
Snapple Teas, 16 oz bottle	13 tsp	50 gm	200 sugar calories
Sprite or 7-up, 12 oz	10 tsp	39 gm	156 sugar calories
Sprite or 7-up, diet, 12 oz	0 tsp	0 gm	0 sugar calories
Sunny D, original flavor, 12 oz	11 tsp	44 gm	176 sugar calories
Starbuck's Frappuccino, Mocha, 13.7 oz bottle	11 tsp	46 gm	186 sugar calories
Starbuck's White Choc Mocha, no whip, nonfat, Grande	15 tsp	59 gm	236 sugar calories
Tang, as prepared, 12 oz	9 tsp	36 gm	144 sugar calories

*Nutrition information provided by www.calorieking.com .

The Amount of Sugar Consumed by the Average American Child Every Two Weeks

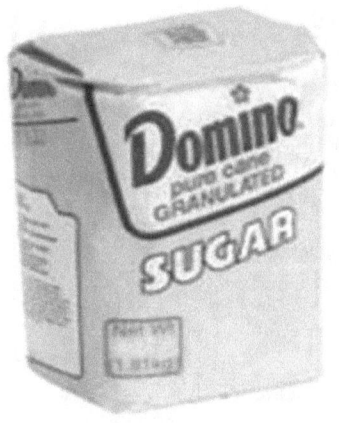 $= 5 \text{ lb.}$

Source: American Diabetes Association

Is the Pyramid Wrong?

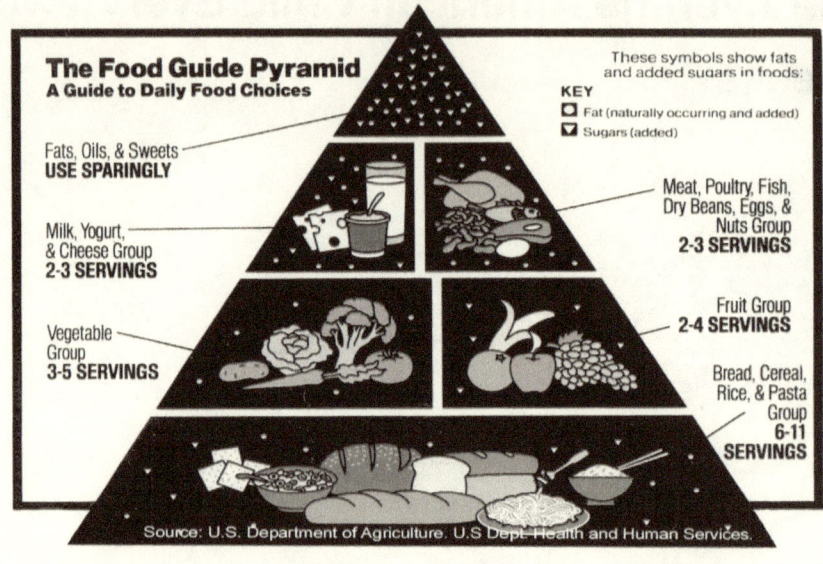

If you look at the small print, the pyramid recommends 6 to 11 servings of starchy foods per day. Each serving = ½ cup or 1 slice of bread.

Typical Serving of Pasta at a Restaurant

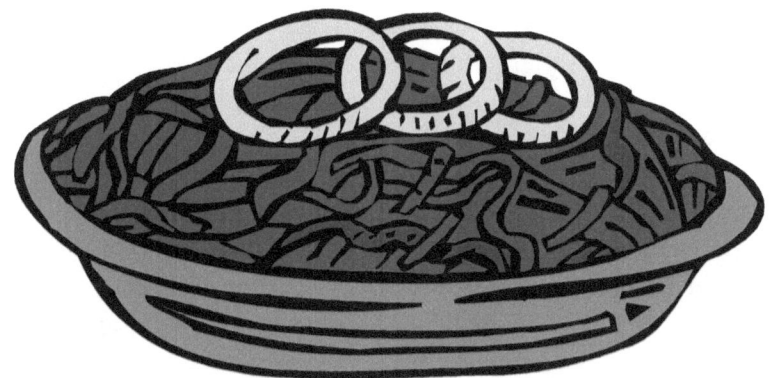

3 ½ cups = 11 starch servings
+ sweetened sauces + bread + sodas
= way too many carbohydrates

5. Repeated Dieting

Some people are surprised to hear me say that dieting is a cause of overweight. I am sure that many of you have heard the adage that "diets don't work". But what, you may ask, is the the rationale for this?

Let us say that your body needs 1800 calories to attain and maintain your body weight. If you go on a weight loss program that provides significantly less than this amount of calories, your metabolism will slow down to the point that it will only burn whatever you are giving it. Also, when people are trying to lose weight, they do so by trying not to eat or to eat less often, both of which also slow the metabolism and reduce the number of calories our body will burn. Then, when we go back to eating the same way we used to eat (ie. go off the diet), we will not only regain the lost weight, but actually gain even more. This is due to the slowing of the metabolism which can occur from eating too little or not often enough.

In his fascinating book, *The Calloway Diet: Starvers, Stuffers, and Skippers* (1990), C. Wayne Calloway, author, researcher, and physician, describes a phenomenon he called cultural-biological dissonance (CBD). He describes that whether a cultural standard desires thinness or plumpness (as in the artist Ruben's time), people will either starve themselves or stuff themselves in an attempt to fit the standard.

Next, biological adaptations will resist these drastic changes in body size and lead to a pattern of repeated failure. Then the failure is attributed to a lack of willpower and self-control, and the person trying to lose (or gain) weight will become fertile ground for exploitive industries that offer to help with special diets, foods, or pills.

So here we are in our American society that idolizes slenderness, yet is by far gaining weight faster than any other on earth.

In the American Dietetic Association's position paper on weight management, they state, "As the environment promotes increased caloric consumption and decreased physical activity, Western culture places a value on attractiveness and interprets slenderness as essential to attractiveness. This interpretation of attractiveness demands conformity to a narrow definition and leaves no room for individual differences. It indicates that those who fail to conform will be denied success, love, power, and other rewards."

God gave us this temple (our body) for which to nourish and care. We were never expected to all look the same. Just as some of us have brown eyes and some blue, we are meant to be different sizes and shapes.

Just as the blue bird does not wish to be a canary, we need to see ourselves as God created us to be. We may not have society's interpretation of the perfect body, but it was given to us by a wonderful and loving God.

Understandably, we may have abused our temple over the years, whether intentional or not, but if we have, He will forgive.

If we were heavy most of our lives, chances are that we were meant to be "more rounded". We need to accept that and encourage the rest of society to accept differences in weight, just as we encourage differences in race. I consider people to judge others based on their weight as "weightists", similar to "racists".

Granted, there are those who have abused our bodies, but from learning how to truly feed our bodies with foods from God's great earth, we will likely lose the excess weight that has come from our societal changes of natural foods.

Some believe that repeated dieting may be responsible for up to one-third of the obesity epidemic in our society, because dieting can make you fat.

Most of my own clients will tell you that they would love to have their previous body back, before they ever started their first diet. They just got bigger and bigger with each successive one.

The way dieting makes us gain weight is by slowing the metabolism (the rate at which we burn calories). In the book mentioned earlier, C. Wayne Calloway would actually measure the metabolisms of his patients using a method called indirect calorimetry. He found that patients who had either been on multiple diets (starvers) or who skipped meals (skippers) were more likely to have a lower metabolism than expected norms and lower than others who did not diet repeatedly or skip meals.

The way the body's metabolism slows down from dieting is as follows: Let's say a person needs 1,600 calories per day to attain their ideal weight. This calorie need is based on a person's age, height, sex, ideal weight, and physical activity level.

Perhaps this person had been overeating and consuming about 2,000 calories per day and decided to go on a weight-loss diet.

Many of the popular diets contain about 1,200 calories per day at most. The body perceives these low-calorie diets as a shortage or deficit and will slow itself down in response to this.

Then when the person stops the diet and goes back to eating the way they did before, the weight piles right back on, but with a few extra pounds because the body is now burning fewer calories.

Again, to repeat our motto:

If it's not a PLAN
You think you CAN (stick with)
JUST DON'T DO IT!

Because if you do, the pounds and your fat cells will just come back and will usually bring a few friends.

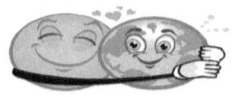 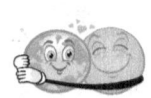 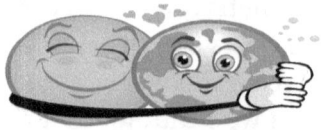

Fat cells before   Fat cells after   Fat cells after-after
weight loss diet   weight loss diet   weight loss diet

Chapter 4

Nature vs. Nurture

(Why Do Some of Us Gain Weight and Get Diabetes Easier Than Others?)

God did not make us to be the same. Just as we were not made to have the same color or texture of hair and skin, we were also not meant to have the same shape of bodies.

Granted, we are seeing a tremendous increase in the rates of obesity, not only in our country, but worldwide. However, if we look at countries where food is in shortage, we will still see rounded people. If we look at prisons, where all prisoners are fed the same and expected to exercise the same, you will still see differences in body shapes.

We are all likely aware of the differences between cultures to be susceptible to various diseases, but were you aware that Native American, Hispanics, African Americans, and Asians have up to ten times the rate of diabetes than Caucasians? Is this because Caucasians eat a healthier diet or exercise more than these more disease-prone people? While it may be true with some, and although these cultures may consume a higher carbohydrate and higher fat diet than Caucasians, lifestyle differences alone do not entirely explain the discrepancies.

Is it possible that the closer our ancestors were to eating natural foods provided by nature, the less able we are to tolerate the processed foods of the Western world?

Evidence for Nature vs. Nurture

Although we do not yet fully understand the exact mechanism for our genetics affecting weight and susceptibility to certain diseases such as diabetes, high blood pressure, and high cholesterol, we are getting closer.

In previous years, there was quite a bit of controversy about whether obesity was affected more by genetics or environment (nature vs. nurture). Of course, it is a combination of the two, but genetics plays a much larger role than many previously believed.

One of the most reliable resources for looking at the subject of weight control is the American Dietetic Association (ADA). To assure accuracy on their Web site, eatright.org, ADA utilizes a group of specially trained dietitians whose job is to "research the research." This group will only consider reviewing research that is performed under the most stringent guidelines. For research to be truly valid and give reliable results, it must pass certain guidelines.

The ADA has a list of position papers that they have written as a result of their extensive research efforts. One of them titled *Weight Management* outlines what the research has found on the genetics and environmental influences on weight control. In this paper, they state that genetic factors account for between 60-80 percent of the predisposition to obesity.

Studies of Twins

Some of the most influential studies have been that of the studies of twins conducted by AJ Stunkard and others in the 1980s and 1990s. These studies looked at pairs of twins who had been reared apart. For instance, they may have been put up for adoption at an early age. Although some of the twins were raised by thin families and other by heavy families, they were much more likely to have body types similar to each other than the families who raised them. Overall, this position paper reports that there are at least several dozen genes that are involved in obesity.

Pima Indians

Another interesting study looking at the strong genetic component of obesity and diabetes is that of the Pima Indians of south-central Arizona. The Pima are modern descendants of the Hohokam people who originated in Mexico.

The Pima Indians settled the land where the Gila and Salt rivers meet in what is now Arizona. They were known as generous people, sheltering peaceful tribes from more hostile tribes. They established a sophisticated system of irrigation that made the arid desert fruitful. They were hospitable to anyone who traveled the Gila River, a main southern route to the Pacific. They were said to have told Kit Carson in 1846, "Bread is to eat, not to sell. Take what you want."

The Pima Indians of today are still giving. For over the past thirty years, the Pima Indians have participated in research conducted by the National Institute of Health (NIH) as well as the National Institute of Diabetes and Digestive and Kidney Disease (NIDDKD).

The reason there is such strong interest in studying these people is their extremely high incidence of obesity and diabetes. Although 6 to 8 percent of the general U.S. population is estimated to have diabetes, the rate of diabetes in the Pima Indians is closer to 40 percent (which jumps to 77 percent of Pima Indians who are older than fifty-five), makes them the most diabetes-prone group of people known to mankind. With a population of over eleven thousand, the willingness of the Pima Indians to participate in this research will help people avoid diabetes; have healthier eyes, hearts, and kidneys; and to understand why people gain weight and what can be done about it. Thanks to this willingness to participate in this research, we now have a much clearer understanding of the genetic predisposition for overweight and diabetes.

Chapter 5

But It is Not All About the Genes . . .

It's Not all Our Genes

Further research has shown that not all is lost if you were born with bad genes. In the 2006 issue of *Diabetes Care*, there was another fascinating study by researchers who compared those Pima Indians of Arizona—that I spoke of back in Chapter 4—with their genetic ancestors, the Pima Indians still living in northern Mexico. The Mexican Pima Indians still live in remote areas only recently accessible by roads and with few modern amenities. Their incidence of diabetes was approximately 7 percent vs. the 40 percent incidence of the Arizona Pima Indians.

Looking at the differences in diet between these two groups, they found that while the Arizona Pima Indians have embraced the more modern Western civilization-style diet (including restaurants such as Taco Bell and KFC), the Mexican Pima Indian diet is relatively low in fat and includes almost no processed foods.

Even though the diet of the Pima Indians still residing in Mexico consists largely of higher carbohydrate foods, such as potatoes and corn tortillas, these were not the processed forms of carbohydrates eaten by the modern Western world. Even the tortillas are generally not the processed kind found in U.S. supermarkets. The Mexican Pima Indians tend to make their tortillas the old-fashioned way, grinding whole dried corn (called stone ground) to make their masa. This is significantly different from our processed packaged tortillas, made either from de-germed corn meal or (even worse) white flour.

In fact, the Mexican Pima Indians were found to consume more than 50 grams of fiber per day, whereas the Arizona Pima Indians ate only 12 to 15 grams per day (as does the average American).

H.H.B.E: Four Top Reasons Why We May Overeat

- **Hunger.** Ask yourself, did you go more than three to four hours between meals? It is important to eat *before* the feelings of hunger hit. By the time these feelings hit, your body is already in the mode for storing whatever it is that you will eat.

  If it was less than three to four hours since your last meal or snack, you may be hungry because of *what* you ate. If it was too high in simple carbohydrates and/or without enough protein, you may find yourself feeling hungry too soon after you eat.
- **Habit.** Do you find yourself eating whenever you sit in front of the TV or computer? When you go out, do you tend to overindulge? Are you in the habit of drinking sodas or high calorie alcoholic beverages? These habits can add up more than we think.
- **Boredom**. If you find yourself eating because you are bored, you may want to find a hobby that requires you to use both of your hands and does not make it easy to eat while doing it. Examples of these would be scrapbooking, knitting, jewelry making, model cars, or tinkering around in the shop.
- **Emotions.** Many of us are emotional eaters. Food, especially high carbohydrate foods, can effect us in a way to that of any addicting substance, such as drugs or alcohol. If you realize that you are unable to kick the high-carb habit on your own, you may reach out to a reputable mental health professional to assist you with proven methods of stress management and problem solving. Another option is Food Addicts (FA). It is a twelve-step approach similar to Alcoholics Anonymous but geared for those whose addiction is food.

Chapter 6

What Is Insulin Resistance (or the Genetic Predisposition for Overweight—GPO)?

We used to think that it was obesity that caused diabetes, hypertension, or high cholesterol. While it may be true that there is a correlation between weight and these diseases, many researches and medical experts now believe that many people are born with a genetic predisposition for gaining weight easily. This condition has been called insulin resistance, metabolic syndrome, or syndrome X. For simplicity's sake, I will just refer to it as insulin resistance and the Genetic Predisposition for Overweight (GPO).

It is estimated that as many as 25 to 50 percent of the American population are predisposed to this condition. If you are of certain ethnic backgrounds, such as Hispanic, African American, Asians, or American Indians, the incidence is even higher.

Personally, I believe that if you see an overweight child, the chances are that he or she has GPO. Chances are, this child has friends who seem to be able to eat whatever they like and do not get much more exercise, but still remain thin. This child likely does not have insulin resistance.

The child with insulin resistance may have other symptoms evident on the body. These may include a dark, thickened, "velvety" skin around the back of the neck and on the knuckles of the hands. This is a condition called Acanthosis Nigricans and is often seen in someone who has insulin resistance. You may also see small pimple-like bumps on the backs of the arms, which is another common symptom of this syndrome.

Let me show you what insulin resistance or GPO looks like using diagrams:

When we eat food, the carbohydrates (starchy foods, such as rice, potatoes, and breads, sweets, fruits, sodas and juices) turn into glucose. This is not necessarily a bad thing, since glucose is the main fuel on which the body runs.

This glucose first enters our bloodstream and, from there, goes into our body's cells.

Two of the main body cells that are fueled by glucose are the muscle cells and the fat cells.

What is Insulin Resistance
also known as Genetic Predisposition for Overweight (GPO)?

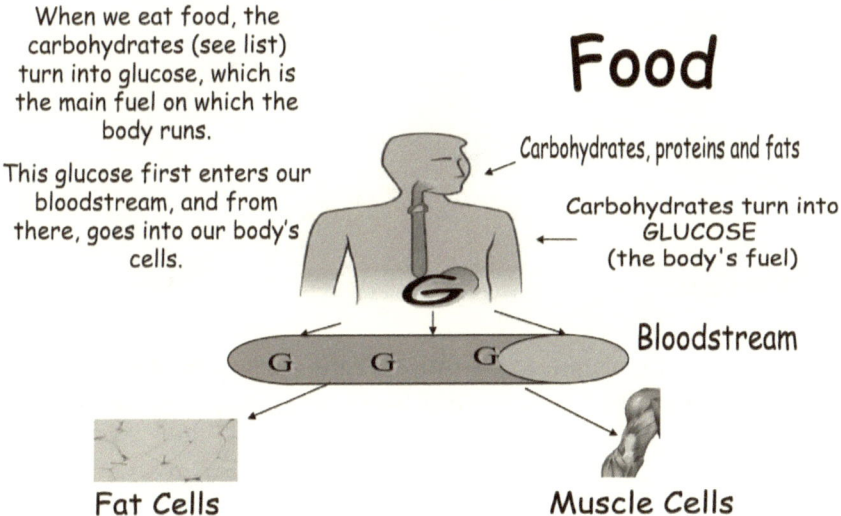

When we eat food, the carbohydrates (see list) turn into glucose, which is the main fuel on which the body runs.

This glucose first enters our bloodstream, and from there, goes into our body's cells.

Food

Carbohydrates, proteins and fats

Carbohydrates turn into GLUCOSE (the body's fuel)

Bloodstream

Fat Cells

Muscle Cells

The hormone insulin (I) is necessary to get the glucose inside the cells. Insulin works like a key to allow the glucose to enter the cells.

Insulin Resistance aka GPO

The hormone Insulin (I) is necessary to get the glucose inside the cells.

Insulin works like a **key** to allow the glucose to enter the cells.

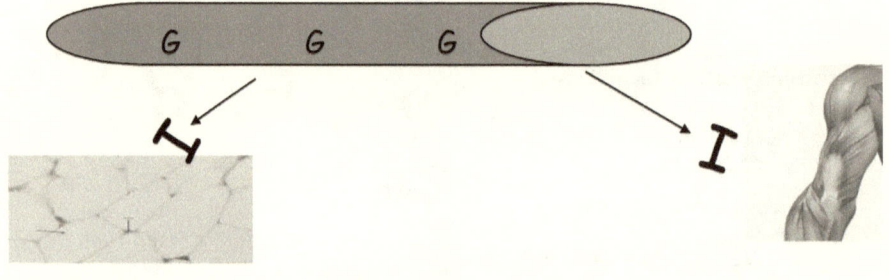

Fat Cells   **Muscle Cells**

With insulin resistance, the muscle cells are resistant to insulin, so the path where the glucose would feed the muscle cells is somewhat blocked.

If the pathway to the muscles cells is somewhat blocked, the glucose is instead going to feed the fat cells.

Insulin Resistance aka GPO

With insulin resistance, the muscle cells are resistant to insulin, so the path where the glucose would feed the muscle cells is somewhat blocked.

If the pathway to the muscles cells is somewhat blocked, the glucose is instead going to feed the fat cells.

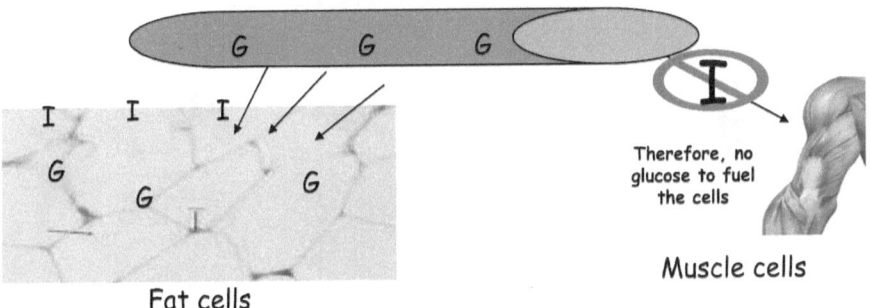

Therefore, no glucose to fuel the cells

Muscle cells

Fat cells

The more carbohydrates we consume in a meal, the more glucose is dumped into our bloodstream. The more glucose in our bloodstream, the more insulin is produced. It is said that someone with insulin resistance will produce more insulin than someone without. This overproduction is known as hyperinsulinemia (too much insulin in the blood).

In people who are insulin resistant, this excess insulin would not get into the muscle cells as it should and would instead allow this excess glucose easy passage to the fat cells.

Therefore in persons with insulin resistance, not only is the problem that the muscle cells are resistant to the insulin, but also that their bodies produce excess insulin in response to carbohydrate intake, which in turn allows for more glucose to be stored in the fat cells.

Insulin Resistance aka GPO

The more carbohydrates we consume in a meal, the more glucose is dumped into our bloodstream. The more glucose in our bloodstream, the more insulin is produced. It is felt that someone with insulin resistance will produce more insulin than someone without. This overproduction is known as hyperinsulemia (too much insulin in the blood).

In people who are insulin resistant, this excess insulin would not get into the muscle cells as it should and would instead allow this excess glucose easy passage to the fat cells.

Therefore in persons with insulin resistance, not only is the problem that the muscle cells are resistant to the insulin, but also that their bodies produce excess insulin in response to carbohydrate intake which in turn allows for more glucose to be stored in the fat cells.

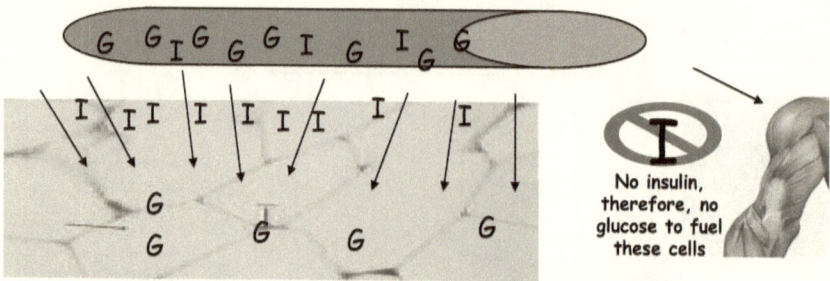

No insulin, therefore, no glucose to fuel these cells

Since the genetic predisposition for obesity (GPO) is a syndrome rather than a disease, it is difficult to diagnose by a single lab test. A fasting insulin level may determine if one has GPO, but more than likely it is a variety of symptoms that leads to a diagnosis, including the following:

High triglycerides

Low HDL (good cholesterol)

High LDL (bad cholesterol)

High blood pressure

Symptoms of low blood sugars (headaches, shakiness, nervousness, irritability, sweating, etc.) that go away after eating

Polycystic Ovary Syndrome (PCOS)

Family history of metabolic syndrome or diabetes

Obesity, especially in younger years

Acanthosis Nigricans (a thick, dark, velvety appearing skin around the neck, knuckles, armpits or inner thighs)

Chapter 7

How to Eat with GPO: General Guidelines

1. **Decrease your carbohydrate intake by limiting or avoiding all processed carbohydrates while continuing to eat natural carbohydrates.** Processed carbohydrates may be useful for feeding masses of people rather cheaply in third world countries with starving people, but are truly not necessary nor recommended in a country such as ours with an abundance of natural foods. As mentioned before, when we eat these processed carbohydrates, they stimulate our insulin levels, cause our bodies to store them very quickly, and then leave us hungry soon after. So instead of that snack of pretzels (white flour), try a few naturally sweet dates and a small handful of nuts.

Limit carbohydrate foods that are PROCESSED

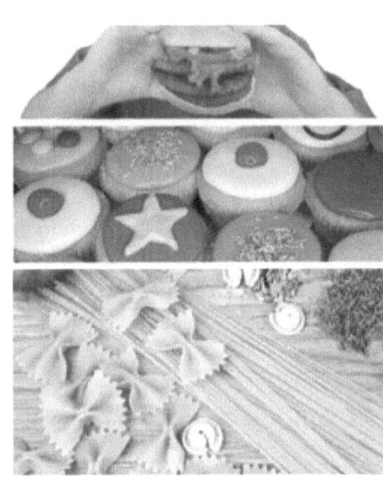

- White flour or white breads
- Processed sugar
- White rice
- White noodles and pasta or noodles
- Juices (processed fruit) (limit to 4 - 8 oz. per day, at most)

It has been estimated that a full 90% of the American food dollar is spent on processed foods.

Choose Instead Natural Carbohydrate Foods:

- Whole grain breads and cereals if you choose to eat these
- Natural sweeteners—very small amounts of honey, stevia, real maple syrup, agave nectar or fruit juice. Sugar substitutes such as Ideal (registered name symbol), Splenda, Equal, or Sweet and Low may also be safely used to provide sweetness with no added calories or carbohydrates, if desired.
- Brown rice and whole wheat pasta (or just significantly limit your serving sizes of the white stuff)
- Starchy vegetables and legumes, such as potatoes, beans, corn, peas, etc.
- Any non-starchy vegetables, such as green beans, carrots, zucchini, artichokes, etc.

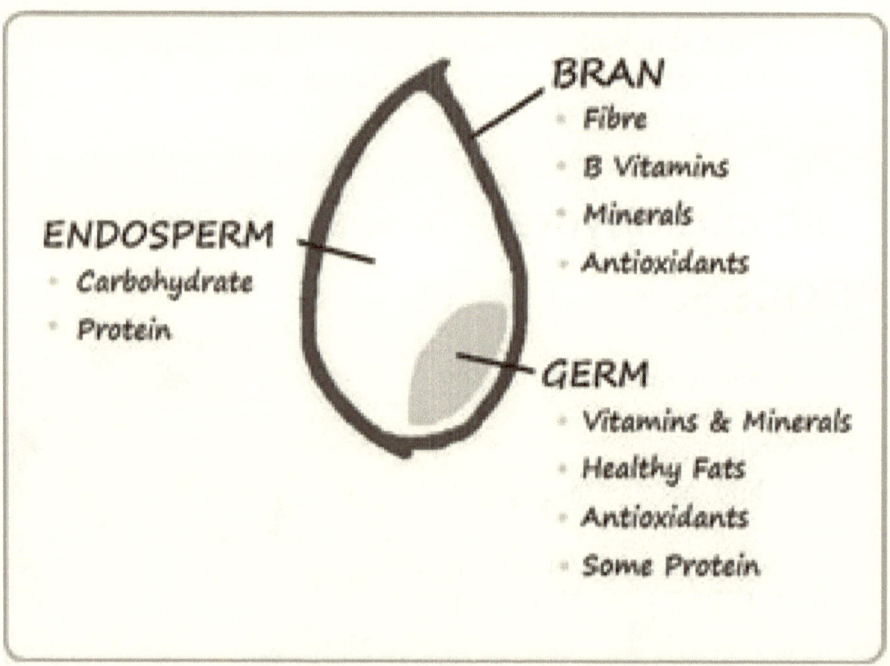

Why is whole grain better than processed grain?

When a grain is processed, the outer covering (the bran layer) is removed. This is were the fiber and a portion of the protein is found.

Next the germ (think wheat germ, not bacteria-type germ) is removed. The removal of the grain germ is the reason for processing the grain, as it contains essential oils. These oils cannot be stored for long period of time without turning rancid (as will all fats), so by removing this germ, the grains can be stored for indefinite periods of time. Unfortunately, this bran layer is where the B-vitamins, vitamin E and other anti-oxidants can be found.

This leaves only the endosperm, which is primarily the starch component. Without the natural bran shell and other essential nutrients, such as adequate protein and fatty acids, to slow down the digestion and absorption, these are assimilated in the body much like pure sugar.

You will notice that most processed grains will contain the word "enriched". This is because it was found that people quickly became deficient in several nutrients when they ate processed grains. Therefore food manufacturers added some of the nutrients back, which is the meaning of the word "enriched". This may have kept people from becoming immediately nutrient depleted, but on a longer range scale, they are causing us to still be deprived of some very essential nutrients. This lack or reduction of nutrients; especially the fiber, essential fatty acids and protein leads to over-eating, as these nutrients are essential to the feeling of fullness (or satiety).

The following diagrams will describe in detail the differences in the nutrient content of a whole grain as compared to one that has been processed.

Comparison of Whole Wheat vs. Unenriched Refined Wheat (similar for other grains as well, such as rice and corn)

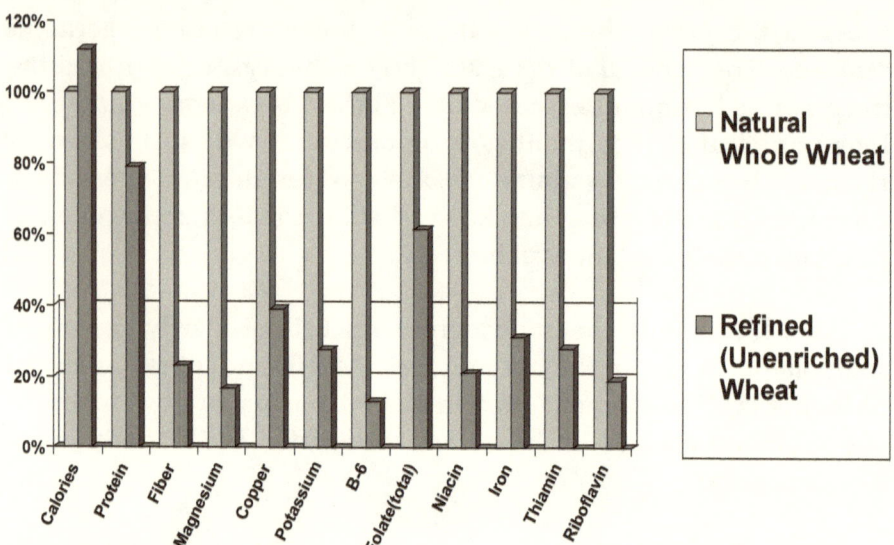

Comparison of Whole Wheat vs. Unenriched Refined Wheat and Enriched Refined Wheat

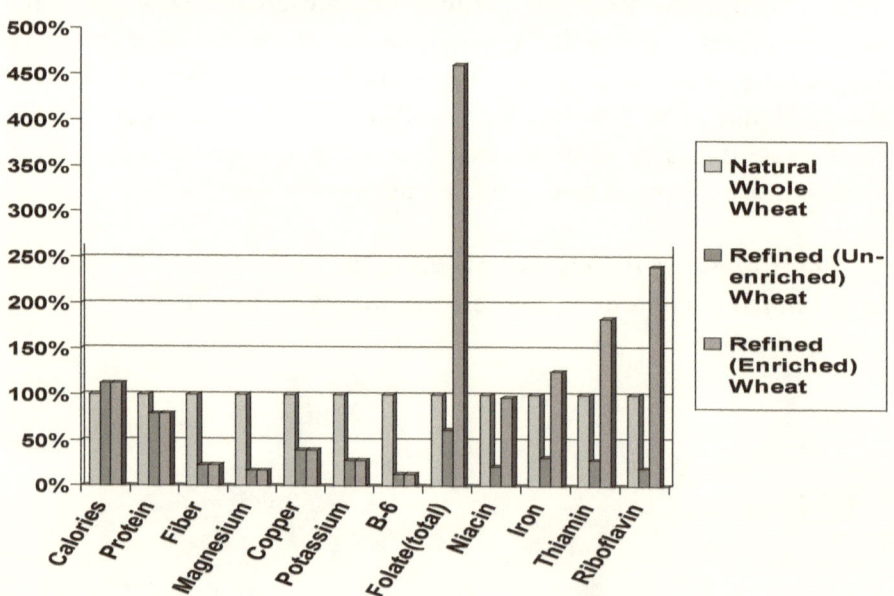

Obviously, enrichment of nutrients may add back some of the nutrients, such as the B-vitamins (some possibly to the level of over-kill), but still does not add back the protein, fiber and several other essential nutrients.

Personally, I prefer not to eat any of those cheap, soft, squishy loaves and rolls some companies try to pawn off as bread. These are made of a mixture that is closer to a foam than a dough. It is stripped of all of it's fiber, most of it's vitamins, then "bleached" with a chemical bleaching compound. How in the world can this be good for us?

Instead, if you choose to eat bread, choose those that are 100% whole grain. To determine if a bread is whole grain, you need to ignore the front of the bread wrapper. Just consider this another advertisement rather than the real story. Instead of looking at the front wrapper, you can turn the bread over and look under the Ingredient part of the label. When reading the ingredients, realize that whatever is listed first has the greatest quantity and it goes down from there. The first word under the Ingredients should be "whole grain", rather than "wheat flour" or "enriched wheat flour".

My daughter once brought home a loaf a bread. The label read "Made with whole wheat", so she thought she was choosing a good bread. On closer review of the label, I discovered that there was actually more high fructose corn sugar in this loaf of bread than whole grain.

Sometimes, breads that are labeled as "wheat bread" are merely white bread with some brown food coloring added. After all, it is wheat, right?

So make sure that if you are eating bread that it is as close to the way God intended as possible. There are even some breads out there that are made by sprouted grains (such as wheat berries, barley, beans, lentils, millet and spelt. In fact, according to the company who makes it, it was inspired by the Holy Scripture verse Ezekiel 4:9., "Take also unto thee Wheat, and Barley, and beans, and lentils, and millet, and Spelt, and put them in one vessel, and make bread of it..."

2.   Replace some of the carbohydrates with protein.

Choose More Natural Protein Sources:

- Natural lean meats, fish, and poultry
- Eggs
- Low-fat cheeses, such as mozzarella or 2 percent cheeses
- Low-fat dairy products, such as 1 percent or nonfat milk
- Low-fat yogurts
- Canadian bacon or ham if you crave breakfast meats
- Nuts and/or nut butters

I generally recommend eating some protein with every meal or snack. Even if you are just eating a natural carbohydrate food, such as fruit, it is good to eat with it some protein. The protein helps to stimulate the hormone that tells the pancreas that it does not need to over-produce the insulin. It is believed that the overproduction of insulin is what leads to the decrease in pancreatic (beta cell) function and ultimately can lead to Type 2 diabetes.

In processed grains, such as white flour, white noodles and/ or white rice), the bran layer (fiber), the germ (healthy oils), several vitamins and protein have been stripped from them. You will notice that these processed grains usually have the word "enriched" associated with them. This is because it was noted that people were becoming quite vitamin deficient when eating these and could die from these deficiencies. Therefore, the food processors added back a few of the vitamins that had been stripped. But they never added back the healthy oils, the fiber or the protein. In my opinion, they are only killing us slower.

While we are in the mode of limiting processed foods, we might as well limit processed meats:

- Hamburger
- Sausage
- Bacon
- Bologna
- Salami
- Pepperoni
- Hotdogs

Try to limit these processed meats to one time per week or less. Most of the processed meats have in them the ground animal fats to help produce bulk and are cheaper to make and sell by the pound. However, these animal fats are saturated and tend to raise our cholesterol levels and clog our arteries. In addition to this, they are usually loaded with added sodium (salt) and contain additives, such as nitrates that can be carcinogenic.

3. <u>Eat smaller, more frequent meals and snacks.</u>

Why are Small, Frequent Meals Important?

While in college, I did some research for my master's degree studying frequency of feeding and the effect on body fat. While looking either at the human or animal studies, I found that if two groups ate the same amount of calories, the group who ate one or two times per day would gain more weight than the group who ate several smaller meals.

1-2 meals per day   **5-6 meals per day**

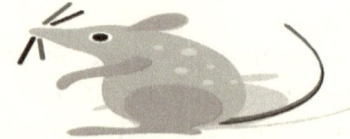   Same number
of calories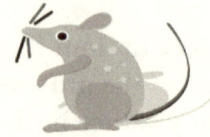

Smaller, more frequent meals are better

There are several possible explanations for this.

First of all, there is a phenomenon called the specific dynamic action of food (SDAF). Whenever we eat (or feed an animal) the body has to go to work to metabolize the food. Therefore, the action of eating and digesting food revs up the metabolism. So if we are to eat five to six times per day versus one to two times per day, it theoretically could increase the amount of calories our body will burn, due to the SDAF.

Not only was this phenomena of eating smaller meals on increasing one's metabolism shown repeatedly with various studies, but newer research is showing that eating only one to two meals per day is correlated to high cholesterol and triglyceride levels as well as heart disease. The body just cannot seem to assimilate a large load of food in one fell swoop with our current sedentary lifestyles.

Let's say that your body can burn off about 1,500 calories per day (or about 500 calories per meal). If you skip breakfast and eat only one to two larger meals, not only will you be hungrier at these meals and likely eat more than your estimated needs, but also, when you eat more calories than your body can metabolize, the difference will be stored. We all know what stored calories look like.

You may figure that you will just burn off the excess calories when you are skipping breakfast the next day, but unfortunately, we do not usually burn fat unless we are doing some form of aerobic exercise.

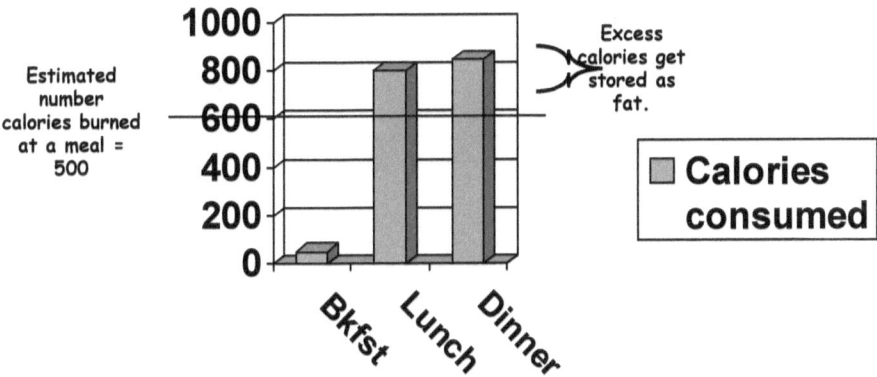

By dividing up your calories into smaller, more frequent meals and snacks, your body is much more likely to be able to utilize the calories for energy and not need to store them.

Please note: When your doctor or other health professional recommends that you add snacks to your diet, some people misinterpret this as adding more calories. But what they really mean is to make the meals smaller and use the calories you saved for between-meal snacks.

In addition to the above reasons for eating smaller meals and snacks, is that we do not want to wait until we get overly hungry before we eat. Although it may sound counter-intuitive, it is better to eat before you get that feeling of extreme hunger.

Not only are you more likely to grab whatever slides down quickly (make less healthy choices), you are also likely to eat a larger volume of food when you start out overly hungry. In addition to this, when you wait until you are extremely hungry to eat and have those feelings that often accompany this (shakiness, headaches, irritability, or lightheaded-ness), your body has begun to release stress hormones. These hormones, epinephrine (adrenaline), norepinephrine, and cortisol start a series of reactions to keep the body from starvation. But they also get the body prepared for storage. Therefore, if you wait too long between meals and/or snacks, your body will store foods more readily.

Think of your metabolism (the amount of calories your body burns) as being like a bonfire. If you want to keep this fire burning, you need to keep throwing logs (small meals and/or snacks) on it.

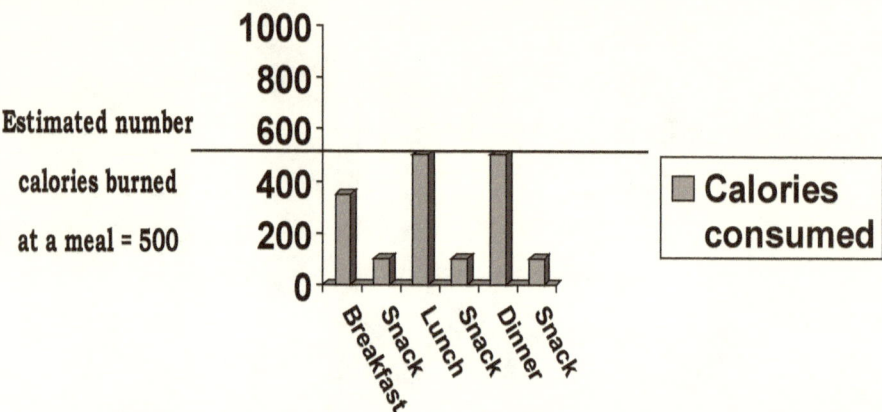

People often think that if they are only eating one or two meals per day, they will burn off their excess fat calories the next day during the time they are not eating. Unfortunately, it doesn't tend to work this way. We generally will not burn excess fat calories unless we are engaging in some form of aerobic exercise.

What will more likely happen is waiting to eat until we are overly hungry, and then we are at risk for making less-than-optimal choices and/or overeating.

In addition to this, when we wait until we are overly hungry before we eat, our body may store what we eat more efficiently. This is especially problematic for those who have insulin resistance.

Here's what tends to happen:

- Wait too long to eat
- Blood sugars drop (hypoglycemia—too little sugar in the blood)
- Body feels hungry, headachy, shaky, or otherwise out of sorts
- Liver and muscle cells release glucose to keep us from starvation
- Blood sugar goes up
- Pancreas releases insulin in response to the rise in blood sugar
- Insulin is a storage hormone.
- Whatever we eat now gets stored (as fat).

4. Increase our movement (exercise) to make our muscle cells more sensitive to the insulin.

As I described in my illustration of insulin resistance, or GPO, the muscle cells seem to be resistant to the hormone insulin. The best way to make these cells become more sensitive to the insulin is by exercise.

Granted, exercise is more difficult if we are massively overweight, but it will along with eating more healthfully, make our bodies feed the muscle cells instead of the fat cells.

Be aware, however, that the muscle cells will be fed, and muscle cells may weigh three times as much as fat cells. Therefore, you may not see as much change in your weight as you would hope to see with exercise, but you should see the change with your clothing sizes, body measurements, or body fat percentage. Try not to use the scale as your only measure of your success while exercising.

Also Extremely Important, Include Fruits and Vegetables

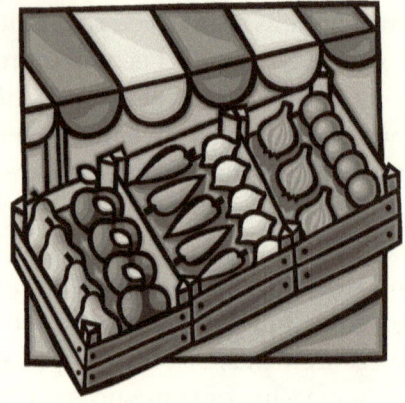

- Nature made them.
- Provide protection mechanisms (such as phytochemicals) for preventing cancers and other chronic diseases.
- We are learning more all the time about their benefits.

Overall, when following the guidelines for eating with GPO, each meal should ideally contain between 30 - 60 gm of carbohydrates. The range depends on a person's size, age, sex and activity level. For instance, a 65 year-old woman who is five feet tall and relatively inactive likely needs closer to 30 gm of carbohydrates per meal, whereas a tall, younger and/or more active person may need 60 gm of carbohydrates (or more).

Then we should try to eat between-meal snacks within 3 - 4 hours of our meals, which should include about 15 - 30 gm of carbohydrates.

Realize, however, that these numbers are merely estimates for the general public. Certain people, such as young athletes, may require much more.

You then want to be sure to include some protein with every meal or snack. As a general rule, I try to get at least one gram of protein for every 2 grams of carbohydrate. For instance, if you eat a fiber bar that contains 22 gm of carbohydrates, it is best if you get at least 11 gm of protein with this bar.

Even when eating natural carbohydrates, such as fruit, it is still good to eat it with some protein (like one ounce of nuts, nut butter, a piece of string cheese or a hard boiled egg). Including the protein with the carbohydrates helps to stimulate the hormone that tells the pancreas that it does not need to over-produce the insulin. It is believed that the overproduction of insulin is what leads to the decrease in pancreatic (beta cell) function and ultimately can lead to Type 2 diabetes.

How Safe Are Artificial Sweeteners?

As you can tell, I am big on natural foods, and obviously, artificial sweeteners are not made by God. But are they safe for those who prefer the sweet taste but cannot seem to tolerate regular processed sugars (such as cane sugar or beet sugar)?

The American Dietetic Association (ADA) is a wonderful source of highly researched information. This is the parent group who oversees registered dieticians. This group has people whose job is to "research the research." They will not even consider using research unless it was conducted under very stringent guidelines, which would deem it valid and reliable research.

This group wrote a position paper on artificial sweeteners. It can be found on their Web site at eatright.org.

Let's Look at Aspartame

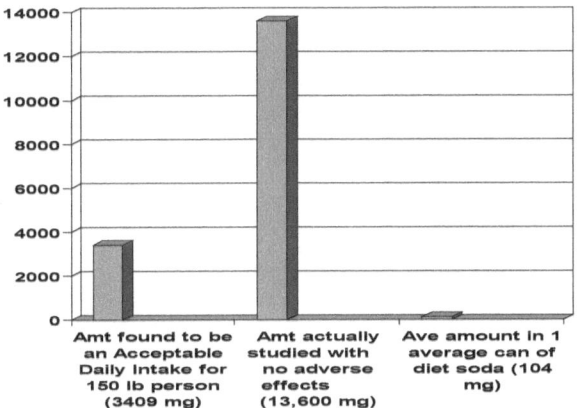

Although aspartame has probably received the most negative press regarding its potential dangers, the American Dietetic Association found it to be safe, even when consumed at levels much greater than usual intakes.

As an aside, I have recently discovered a new sweetener made by Heartland Sweeteners® called Ideal® No Calorie Sweetener. It is made with Xylitol, which is a naturally occurring sugar alcohol that can be found in many fruits and vegetables and is even produced by the human body as part of the normal metabolism of glucose. With its low glycemic index, xylitol is great for people with diabetes since it is metabolized independently of insulin. AND IT TASTES TRULY GREAT!

Making it simple to eat with GPO

Instead of eating meals that are primarily processed carbohydrates, such as pasta, make an effort to make your plate a little more balanced using this diagram as a simple guide:

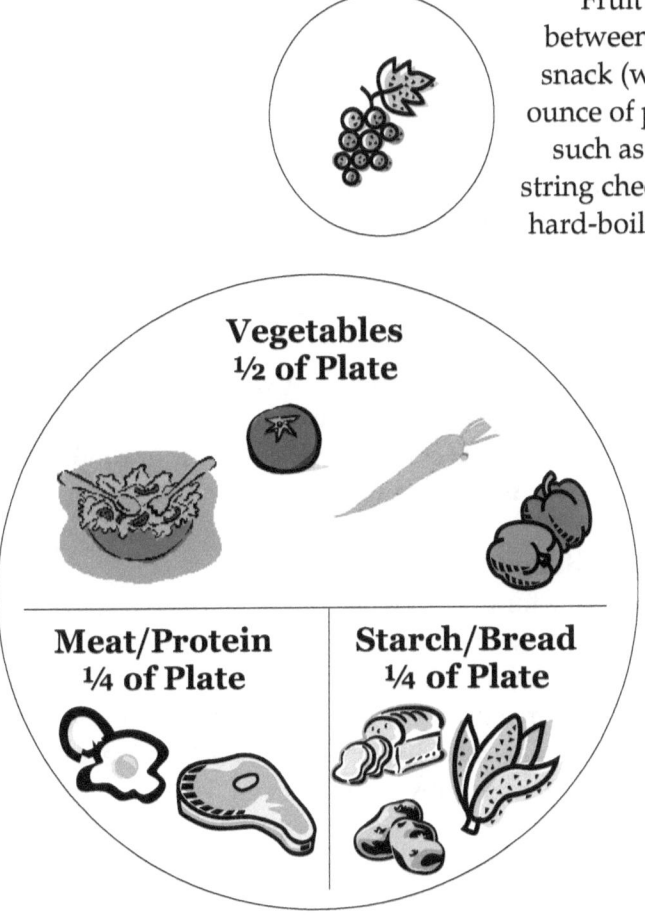

Fruit for between-meal snack (with an ounce of protein, such as nuts, string cheese, or a hard-boiled egg)

Vegetables
½ of Plate

Meat/Protein
¼ of Plate

Starch/Bread
¼ of Plate

Chapter 8

Stage One of the Diet of Eden: The Carb Cleanse

Note: Check with your physician before starting this plan, especially if you are a diabetic and taking insulin or pills that can cause your blood sugars to drop too low.

Also, it is very important that you do not try to maintain this reduced carbohydrate meal plan for more than two weeks. As mentioned earlier in the book, the body is meant to be maintained with a balance of carbohydrates, fats and proteins. If we remove too many carbohydrates for a long period of time, the diet would then be either too high in fats or proteins. Neither of these would be healthy long term. Therefore it is important that you be sure to include the natural carbohydrates (starchy vegetables, fruits, whole grains) back into your diet after the two week cleanse.

Optional Carbohydrate Cleansing Plan:
It is not necessary for everyone to complete this part of The Diet of Eden. For instance, if your diet is already relatively low in processed carbohydrates, then stage one is likely not necessary for you. However, if you feel that if you are currently eating a diet that is full of processed carbohydrates, this stage may be for you. There are several reasons you may want to try the carbohydrate cleanse:

1. It makes you more aware where the carbohydrates are in your diet.
2. It makes you realize that, while it is not easy, it is possible to live without all of these processed carbohydrates. PLEASE NOTE: I DO NOT RECOMMEND TRYING TO STAY WITH THIS LOWER LEVEL OF CARBOHYDRATES FOR A LONGER THAN TWO WEEKS AT A TIME. Carbohydrates are to the body as gas is to a car: the fuel that

it runs on. They are also the most efficient form of energy for the body. Also, by trying to stick with the lowered levels of carbohydrates outlined in the Carb Cleanse, most people will eventually begin to feel cheated, and not be able to stick with it.

3. It makes you appreciate the natural carbohydrates once they are added back to the diet.

It is important that you follow the recommendations of including each day:

- ❑ **2 (8 oz.) cups per day of milk, soy milk, and/or plain or light yogurt. (may contain small bits of fruit)**
- ❑ **½-1 cup of legumes (beans, such as kidney beans, garbanzos, pinto beans, etc.) Note: canned beans are acceptable here.**
- ❑ **If you choose not to eat beans, then you will need to eat an additional cup of milk or light yogurt each day.**

Other than these important recommendations, you may enjoy unlimited amounts* of the foods in the left hand column and avoid (for two weeks) the foods on the right hand column.

* You may notice that nuts are limited to ⅓ cup at a time. You may eat them more than once per day, but keep the portion to ⅓ cup.

Are You Ready for the First Fourteen Days?

(Do you have the items on hand?)

Enjoy
(unlimited unless otherwise indicated)

Lean Meats or Proteins

Note: Be sure to include the first two items on this list daily.

❑ Milk, plain soy milk or yogurt (plain or light [low sugar])—limit to 2 cups per day for first fourteen days.

❑ Beans: pinto, garbanzo, lentils, navy, kidney—limit to ½-1 cup per day for first fourteen days. If unable to eat the beans, you may include one extra cup of milk or light yogurt.

❑ Lean beef such as ground round, tenderloin, sirloin, round, flank, cubed, porterhouse, roasts such as chuck, rib, or rump, jerky (with 5 gm carbs or less)

❑ Poultry without skin (chicken, Cornish hen, or turkey)

❑ Pork, lean such as Canadian bacon, rib or loin chop/roast, ham, tenderloin

❑ Fish (canned or fresh)

❑ Shellfish such as clams, crab, imitation shellfish, lobster, scallops, shrimp

❑ Cheese

❑ Cottage cheese

❑ Eggs or egg substitute

❑ Peanut butter

❑ Tofu

❑ Nuts (keep portions to ⅓ cup)

Avoid for fourteen days

High Fat Meats and Proteins

❑ High fat, processed meats,
❑ such as sausage, bacon, salami, pepperoni, and regular hotdogs.

❑ Spareribs

❑ Any meats made with sweet sauces, such as teriyaki sauce, sweet and sour sauce, barbeque sauce or ketchup.

Enjoy (unlimited)	Avoid for fourteen days

■ Any nonstarchy vegetables made by our Lord (including, but not limited to):

- ❑ Asparagus
- ❑ Artichokes
- ❑ Artichoke hearts
- ❑ Baby corn
- ❑ Bamboo shoots
- ❑ Beans (green, wax, Italian)
- ❑ Bean sprouts
- ❑ Beets (unless pickled)
- ❑ Borscht
- ❑ Broccoli
- ❑ Brussels sprouts
- ❑ Cauliflower
- ❑ Cabbage
- ❑ Carrots
- ❑ Celery
- ❑ Cucumber
- ❑ Eggplant
- ❑ Green onions or scallions
- ❑ Greens (collard, kale, mustard, or turnip)
- ❑ Hearts of palm
- ❑ Jicama
- ❑ Kohlrabi
- ❑ Leeks
- ❑ Lettuce
- ❑ Mixed veggies (without corn, peas, or pasta)
- ❑ Mushrooms
- ❑ Okra
- ❑ Onions
- ❑ Pea pods
- ❑ Peppers (all varieties)
- ❑ Radishes
- ❑ Rutabaga
- ❑ Sauerkraut
- ❑ Spinach
- ❑ Squash (summer, crookneck, zucchini)
- ❑ Swiss chard
- ❑ Tomatoes
- ❑ Tomatoes, canned
- ❑ Tomato/vegetable juice
- ❑ Turnips
- ❑ Water chestnuts

■ Starchy vegetables such as:

- ❑ Cassava
- ❑ Corn
- ❑ Hominy
- ❑ Lima beans
- ❑ Parsnips
- ❑ Peas
- ❑ Plantain, ripe
- ❑ Potatoes
- ❑ Pumpkin
- ❑ Winter squash (acorn, butternut)
- ❑ Yam, sweet potato

■ All breads, rolls, muffins, chapatti, tortillas, etc.
■ All cereals
■ All chips
■ All crackers
■ All rice
■ All pasta
■ All grains, such as barley, millet, quinoa
■ Pancakes
■ Popcorn
■ All fruits (fresh or dried)
■ All juices with 5 gm. or more sugars per serving

Enjoy (unlimited)

- **Beverages**

  - ❑ Water (best)
  - ❑ Herbal tea
  - ❑ Black, green or oolong tea
  - ❑ Coffee (reg. or decaf.)
  - ❑ Propel
  - ❑ Any beverages with 0-5 gm carbohydrates per serving
  - ❑ Diet sodas
  - ❑ Crystal Light
  - ❑ Kirkland Vita-Ice
  - ❑ Diet Kool-Aid
  - ❑ 1 oz. juice mixed with 11 oz. water
  - ❑ Make your own sodas with sparkling water and flavored sugar-free Torani syrups.

- **Miscellaneous***

  (Note: many sugar-free products may contain sugar alcohols (mannitol, sorbitol, etc.) with may cause intestinal gassiness and/or diarrhea).

  - ❑ Sugar-free Popsicles*
  - ❑ Sugar-free Jell-O
  - ❑ Sugar-free Fudgsicles*
  - ❑ Sugar-free candies (up to 100 calories per day)*
  - ❑ Whipping cream
  - ❑ Salsa
  - ❑ Sugar-free chocolate syrup*
  - ❑ Salad dressings and other fats except those listed on the "avoid" list:

    - ▪ Mayonnaise
    - ▪ Ranch
    - ▪ Caesar
    - ▪ Blue cheese
    - ▪ Italian
    - ▪ Vinaigrette
    - ▪ Oil and vinegar
    - ▪ Butter

Avoid

- **Beverages**

  - ❑ Regular sodas
  - ❑ Regular juices
  - ❑ Any beverages with more than 5 gm. carbohydrates per serving
  - ❑ Smoothies
  - ❑ Flavored coffees or teas with more than 5 gm. carbohydrates per serving.
  - ❑ Any alcohol for the first fourteen days

- **Miscellaneous**

  - ❑ Sweet salad dressings such as Thousand Island, French, sweet and sour, honey mustard, etc.
  - ❑ Sugar-free puddings

Menu Ideas for first fourteen days (may repeat any meal or snack as desired):

Breakfast	Snack	Lunch	Snack	Dinner	Snack
Omelet Coffee (cream and artificial sugar)	1 oz. nuts (approx. ¼ cup)	Large chef salad Dressing 8 oz. milk	Low-sugar yogurt	Homemade soup with beans and meat	2 sugar-free Popsicles
High-protein shake with 5 gm sugar or less	Hot tea Fresh veggies Cheese	Meat Salad Veggies	Sugar free Jell-O with whipped cream	Large Caesar chicken salad	Hot herbal tea ⅓ cup nuts
Cottage cheese with tomatoes	Low-sugar yogurt	Protein-style burger (wrapped in lettuce)	1-2 tbsp. peanut butter	Chinese food made with meat/chicken and veggies only (no sweet sauces)	Hot chocolate made with sugar free Hershey's syrup
Leftover meat and veggies	Cottage cheese	Inside of a taco salad (no shell)	1 cup milk with sugar free syrup	Omelet with ham, cheese, and veggies	Sugar free Jell-O with whipped cream
Egg salad over lettuce or deviled eggs Crystal Light	Celery with peanut butter	Homemade soups made with meats and nonstarchy veggies	Fresh veggies with dip Sugar-free beverage	Meat, fish, poultry or cheese Lots of nonstarchy veggies	Sugar-free Fudgsicle
Low-sugar Yogurt ⅓ cup nuts	Protein bar with 5 gm carbohydrates or less	Large salad with eggs, meat, and kidney beans/Dsg	⅓ cup nuts Fresh veggies	Soup made with nonstarchy veggies and meat or chicken	Celery with peanut butter 8 oz. milk
Scrambled eggs with ham Coffee or tea	Veggies with dip Sugar-free beverage	Large Wendy's Chili w/Onions & Cheese	Sugar-free hot chocolate	Salmon Lots of nonstarchy veggies Salad	Cottage cheese with tomatoes

73

Chapter 9

Stage Two: The Natural Carb Plan "The Diet of Eden"

On the following pages, I have outlined a month of menu ideas. These are not perfectly fitting of all of the principles of The Diet of Eden, but they are a start. I have kept some processed carbohydrates in because I do not expect people to give up all of these foods at once. In addition, I needed to consider availability of foods. I realize that not all of us have the time to hand make and pack every single meal and snack, so these first menus are a start. For many people, it is enough of a change to make significant improvements to their health.

For those who are purists, "you may choose to eat" only foods which have been provided in their purest forms by God.

Remember, learning new habits is a journey. Give yourself time to enjoy the journey and do not chastise yourself if you stumble a little in the beginning.

Month of Healthy Breakfast (Try to eat within two hours of waking)

Then include a healthy snack or another small meal every three to four hours

Breakfast casserole[1] ½ Whole grain English muffin Fruit Coffee or tea or other Zero-carbohydrate beverage	Cottage cheese and pineapple 1 slice whole grain toast with small amount of butter Zero-carbohydrate beverage	Quesadilla: whole wheat, stone ground corn or low-carbohydrate tortilla with low-fat cheese and salsa Fresh fruit Zero-carbohydrate beverage	Whole grain, unsweetened cereal 1 tsp. raw sugar 1% or nonfat milk Zero-carbohydrate beverage
French toast sticks with strawberries and almonds[3] Ham or Canadian bacon Zero-carbohydrate beverage	Light yogurt (about 100 calories) 1-2 tbsp. Granola, Grape-Nuts, or Trail Mix Zero-carbohydrate beverage	Low-carbohydrate, high-protein bar (Zone, Balance Bar, Atkins) Zero-carbohydrate beverage	100% whole grain toast with natural peanut butter and all-fruit jam 8 oz. milk Zero-carbohydrate beverage
Breakfast burrito[5] on whole grain or Low-carbohydrate tortillas Low-carbohydrate beverage	Whole grain toaster waffle (such as Kashi®) with peanut butter and small amount of natural maple syrup 8 oz. milk	10-12 Wheat Thins or Rye Crisp crackers Low-Fat cheese Fresh fruit Low-carbohydrate beverage	Whole wheat or low-carbohydrate tortilla with natural peanut butter and all-fruit jam, cut into wedges 8 oz. milk
Purchased low-carbohydrate, high-protein drink Beef or turkey jerky Fresh fruit	½ whole wheat bagel with cream cheese and smoked salmon Fresh fruit Low-carbohydrate beverage	Ham or turkey roll-up in low-carbohydrate tortillas Fresh fruit Low-carbohydrate beverage	Yogurt smoothie[6]
Egg salad on whole grain crackers Fresh fruit Zero-carbohydrate beverage	Starbucks Turkey Bacon, low-fat cheese, and egg sandwich on whole grain English muffin Low-carbohydrate beverage	Homemade high-protein smoothie[2]	Old-fashioned or steel-cut oats ¼ cup raisins or Trail Mix 8 oz. milk Zero-carbohydrate beverage
Half of whole grain bagel Laughing Cow cheese Fresh fruit Zero-carbohydrate beverage	English muffin pizza[4] 8 oz. milk Low-carbohydrate beverage	Lean cold cut sandwich on whole grain bread (sodium-nitrate free, if possible) Piece of fruit Low-carbohydrate beverage	Low-carbohydrate, high-protein shake (Atkins, Glucerna, Costco's Premier Protein, etc.)
Cantaloupe half stuffed with cottage cheese 1 slice whole grain toast w/ small amount butter Low-carbohydrate beverage	6 graham cracker squares spread with natural peanut or almond butter 8 oz milk	½ cup purchased hummus and 1 whole wheat pita or naan Piece of fruit Low-carbohydrate beverage	(Restaurant) Omelet made with vegetables and cheese potatoes Fresh fruit Low-carbohydrate beverage

Month of Healthy Lunches
Include a healthy snack or small meal every three to four hours

Peanut butter and low-sugar jelly Sandwich on whole grain bread Low-sugar (light) yogurt Veggie sticks Zero-carbohydrate beverage	Low-fat cheese and 1 cup fruit 20 Sun Chips Small salad Zero-carbohydrate beverage	Veggie soup ½ cheese Sandwich on whole grain Natural apple sauce Zero-carbohydrate beverage	Chicken salad and 12 whole grain crackers Carrot sticks (8) 1 cup of grapes Zero-carbohydrate beverage
Minestrone soup Peanut butter stuffed in celery Pear Zero-carbohydrate beverage	Tuna sandwich on whole wheat with lettuce & tomato Cucumber slices ½ cup canned fruit	Shrimp cocktail 6 whole grain crackers Large salad Cup of soup Fruit salad Zero-carbohydrate beverage	6" sub sandwich Piece of fruit Zero-carbohydrate beverage
1 chicken taco 1 bean tostada with extra lettuce, tomatoes, and guacamole Diet soda or ice tea	Mexican roll-ups Low-carbohydrate or whole wheat tortilla Veggie sticks Zero-carbohydrate beverage 2 cookies	30 gram or less frozen dinner (Healthy Choice) salad (light on dressing) Pieces of fruit or 2 cookies Zero-carbohydrate beverage	Egg salad on whole wheat 10-12 crackers Fruit Veggies Zero-carbohydrate beverage
Purchased high-protein drink and 5 pieces of beef jerky fruit Zero-carbohydrate beverage	2 pieces veggie Pizza Salad bar Diet soda	Leftover meat loaf, mashed potatoes with gravy Green beans Zero-carbohydrate beverage 2 cookies	Roast beef (sodium nitrate-free) sandwich with lettuce, tomato, and onion Salad (light on the dressing) and Fruit
Lean (sodium nitrate-free) cold cut (roast beef, ham, turkey) or cheese on whole wheat melba toast or rye crisp crackers Tomato soup 1 cup fresh berries	Cottage cheese with ½ cup pineapple 6 Wheat Thins Tomato wedges 2 cookies Zero-carbohydrate beverage	(Out) Grilled chicken sandwich on whole grain bun, wrapped in lettuce, or eat ½ bun only Salad Piece of fruit (small) Zero-carbohydrate beverage	Salad with cheese and nuts Avocado and tomatoes 10-12 whole grain crackers ½ cup canned fruit Zero-carbohydrate beverage
Chicken salad in a whole wheat pita pocket with lettuce (2 halves) Veggie sticks 2 cookies Zero-carbohydrate beverage	2 slices thin crust pizza Large salad (go easy on the dressing) Zero-carbohydrate beverage	Bean soup 4-6 whole grain crackers ½ sandwich on whole grain bread Veggies Zero-carbohydrate beverage	Leftovers 2 pieces of chicken 1 medium potato, cut up Cooked veggies Zero-carbohydrate beverage
Chef salad (light on the dressing) 4-6 whole grain crackers Sugar-free (light) yogurt Zero-carbohydrate beverage	Grilled chicken or fish ⅔ cup Brown rice Vegetables Zero-carbohydrate beverage 2 cookies	Purchased salad (1 cup) String cheese 4-6 Whole grain crackers Zero-carbohydrate beverage Sugar-free Jell-O	Chinese food, but limit rice or noodles to ⅔ cup (lots of veggies & meat or eat with extra veggies and no noodles or rice) Zero-carbohydrate beverage

Month of Healthy Dinners

Roasted Salmon with Lemons & Capers[7] Salad with vinaigrette dressing[8] Veggie of choice Whole wheat Couscous[9] Zero-carbohydrate beverage	Bean soup[10] Whole grain crackers or melba toast Cottage cheese and Fruit salad Zero-carbohydrate beverage	Whole grain pasta (try Barilla Plus) Pasta sauce (find one with the lowest carbohydrates or make your own)[11] Cooked veggies Salad Zero-carbohydrate beverage	Quesadillas made with stone ground corn or flour tortillas[12] Salsa Fresh cut-up veggies Zero-carbohydrate beverage
Garden burgers (store-bought) on whole grain buns with lettuce, tomato, onions, and assorted condiments. Sun Chips	Banana-nut whole grain pancakes[13] Turkey bacon or veggie bacon (fake-un)	Southwestern Soup with Hominy and Pinto Beans[14] Quesadillas made with stone ground corn flour tortillas or low-carbohydrate tortillas Zero-carbohydrate beverage	Taco salad[15] Sugar-free Jell-O with fruit and whipped cream Zero-carbohydrate beverage
Whole grain cheese ravioli with artichoke hearts and pesto[16] Salad Zero-carbohydrate beverage	Super Simple Talapia[17] Corn on the cob Green beans Zero-carbohydrate beverage	Easy Red Beans & Rice[18] Breaded frozen okra Zero-carbohydrate beverage	Frozen dinner (Healthy Choice, Amy's, stone ground etc.) Veggie of choice Salad of choice Zero-carbohydrate beverage
Turkey Burgers with Blue Cheese & Hot Sauce[19] Baby carrots and celery strips Zero-carbohydrate beverage	Artichoke, tomato, and spinach pizza[20] Caesar salad (or salad of choice) Zero-carbohydrate beverage	Fish tacos with mango slaw[21] Black beans Zero-carbohydrate beverage	Simple Homemade Chili[22] Broiled cheese toasts[30] Glass of milk or zero-carbohydrate beverage
Beef stew[23] Side of extra veggies or salad Whole grain bread or roll Zero-carbohydrate beverage	Frozen Veggie pizza on whole grain or thin crust Ready-made salad Zero-carbohydrate beverage Sugar-free Jell-O with a dollop of whipped cream	Crab cakes[24] Roasted Sweet Potatoes[25] Cooked veggies and/ or salad Zero-carbohydrate beverage	Chicken Stir Fry over brown rice [26] Blueberries in lightly sweetened cream[27]
Sloppy Joe's on Whole Grain buns or sandwich "rounds"[28] Carrot sticks Sugar-free pudding	Chef salad[29] Broiled cheese toasts[30] Zero-carbohydrate beverage	Oven "Fried" Chicken[31] Mashed New Red Potatoes[32] Broiled Asparagus with garlic[33] Zero-carbohydrate beverage	Multilayer Mexicali dip[34] stone ground tortilla chips Zero-carbohydrate beverage
Grilled cheese sandwich on whole wheat bread Tomato soup Zero-carbohydrate beverage	Grilled steak Baked potato Spinach Salad Zero-carbohydrate beverage	Smoked Salmon and Chive Omelette[35] Sliced Tomatoes Zero-carbohydrate beverage Sugar-free chocolate pudding with whipped cream	Spaghetti Carbonara[36] Salad of choice Zero-carbohydrate beverage

RECIPES

1. **Breakfast Casserole (serves 4)**
   Preheat oven to 375o. Spray 8" by 8" baking pan with nonstick spray. Pour ½ bag of Ore Ida O'Brien Potatoes (hash browns with onions & peppers) into prepared pan, breaking up large chunks. Cut up 2 oz of ham, Canadian bacon, or lowfat smoked sausage. Sprinkle meat and ½ c. low fat cheddar cheese over potatoes. Whip 2 whole eggs and 4 egg whites, 2 Tbsp milk, 2 Tbsp Dijon mustard and ¼ tsp. thyme. Pour evenly over potatoes. Sprinkle lightly with freshly ground pepper to taste. Place in oven (uncovered) and bake for 40 minutes. Let cool 5 minutes before serving.

2. **High Protein Smoothie (serves 1)**
   Pour 1 cup non fat, 1% or soy milk into blender. Add 1 cup berries or ½ cup canned fruit in juice. Add ¼ container of soft tofu or ¼ cup dry milk powder. Add 2 Tbsp. sugar free Torini flavored syrup (vanilla or strawberry is good) or 1-2 packets Splenda or other sweetener. Add 1 cup crushed ice and blend until smooth.

3. **French Toast Sticks with Strawberries & Almonds (serves 1)**
   Cut one slice of whole grain bread into 4 strips. Beat 1 whole egg and 3 egg whites (or ½ c. egg substitute) till frothy. Spray skillet with non-stick spray. Soak bread in eggs and place in pan over medium heat until lightly browned. (Scramble any remaining eggs to eat with French toast). After cooked, place toast sticks on a plate and sprinkle lightly with powdered sugar. Add 1 cup of strawberries and 1 Tbsp slivered almonds. Serve with bacon on the side.

4. **Yogurt Smoothie (serves 1)**
   Empty one 6-8 oz container sugar-free, fruit flavored yogurt into blender. Add 4 oz tofu or ¼ cup nonfat dry milk. Add ½ cup juice and ice, if desired. Blend until smooth.

5. **English Muffin Pizza (serves 1)**
   Separate one whole wheat English muffin into halves. Spread with pizza sauce, spaghetti sauce or tomato paste. Sprinkle with 2 ounces (1/4 c) mozzarella cheese. Place in broiler about 1 minute or until cheese is melted and lightly browned.

6. **Egg Beater® Breakfast Burrito or Taco**
(serves 1) Cook scrambled egg substitute in lightly oiled pan until firm. Add chilis, tomatoes, olives, peppers, and/or salsa as desired. Serve on 2 small (6 inch) wheat or corn tortillas.

7. **Roasted Salmon with Lemon and Capers**
4 skinless salmon filets, about 6 oz each
4 tsp capers
Juice of 1 lemon
Salt & Pepper

Preheat oven to 450°F. Place salmon on baking sheet. Lightly salt and pepper. Roast salmon about 8 – 10 mins until opaque throughout. Remove from oven. Top each filet with 1 tsp capers and approximately 1 tsp. lemon juice.

8. **Vinegarette Dressing**
1/3 c. vinegar (your choice: balsamic, red wine, cider, etc)
1/3 c. oil
1/3 c. water
1 tsp Italian seasoning
1 clove garlic, chopped fine
Salt and Pepper to taste

Mix all ingredients; store leftover dressing in refrigerator up to one week.

9. **Whole Wheat Couscous**
Cook according to package directions. For liquid, may use water, broth or low sodium broth.

10. **Bean Soup (serves 4)**
(May use a canned version if desired; preferably a lower salt version, such as Health Valleytm.)
To make your own:
1 lb dried navy beans
1 Tbsp olive oil
1 small onion, finely chopped
1 large carrot, sliced

1 stalk celery, sliced
Salt & Pepper to taste
Ham hock, optional.

Rinse beans and place in a pot with 4 cups water. Bring to a boil, turn off heat and allow to sit for 1 hour. Drain beans in colander. While beans are draining, place oil in the pot and cook onions, carrots and celery until just beginning to get tender (about 3 minutes). Add beans to pot and approximately 8 cups of water. Add ham hock, if desired. Cook bean soup for approximately 1-1/2 hour or until beans are tender. After beans are tender, add salt and pepper to taste. Note: Adding salt to the beans before they are cooked my result in tough beans.

11. Homemade Pasta Sauce (serves 4)

1/2 pound lean hamburger, ground turkey or vegetarian meat substitute
1 Tbsp. oil, if needed (If meat or substitute is too lean)
1 medium onion, finely chopped
2 cloves garlic, chopped
2 Tbsp Italian seasoning
Salt and pepper to taste.
1 29oz can tomato sauce
1 6oz can tomato paste
1 cup red wine or water

Cook beef, turkey or meat substitute with onion and garlic until meat is cooked through. Add seasoning. Add the tomato sauce, tomato paste and wine or water. Simmer or very low heat approximately 1 hour.

12. Quesadillas (serves 1)

One 12" or (2) 6" whole grain flour or stone-ground corn tortillas
2 oz (1/4 cup) Low fat Monterey Jack or Cheddar cheese

In a nonstick skillet, heat a small amount of the cheese until slightly melted. Top with tortilla and rest of cheese. Once cheese is completely melted, fold over tortilla (if using 12") or top with 2nd tortilla (if using 6". Flip tortilla and slightly brown other side. Serve with salsa and lower fat sour cream, if desired.

13. Whole Grain Banana Nut Pancakes (makes 4 servings)
2 eggs, beaten
2 ripe bananas, mashed
2 cups white whole wheat flour
½ tsp. nutmeg
2 cups milk
3 Tbsp. butter, melted or oil
2 Tbsp. Idealtm sugar substitute
2 Tbsp. baking powder
½ tsp. salt
¼ cup walnuts or pecans, chopped or ¼ cup hemp hearts

Mix eggs and banana; beat in remaining ingredients and mix just until smooth (do not over-mix). Grease heated griddle. (To test griddle, carefully sprinkle with few drops water. If bubbles skitter around, heat is just right.)

Pour about ¼ cup of batter onto heated griddle. Cook pancakes until puffed and dry around edges. Turn and cook other side until golden brown.

14. Southwestern Soup with Hominy and Pinto Beans
1 Tbsp. Olive Oil
One medium onion, chopped
1 package vegetarian Choriso Sausage (Soyriso®) or Turkey Sausage

Cook onion and sausage until onions are tender and slightly browned.

Add:
8 cups water
1 large can of tomatoes (chopped or pureed)
1 small can tomato paste
1 small can Mexican tomato sauce

1 large can hominy
2 cans pinto Beans

Cook approximately 45 minutes until flavors are well blended.

15. Taco Salad
4 cups shredded lettuce
2 cups (8 oz) lowfat cheddar cheese
3 green onions, sliced (white and green parts)
Small can sliced black olives (optional)
1 tomato, diced
Optional: Coarsely broken tortilla chips, preferably stone ground (about 20)

Dressing:
1 cup sour cream (regular, low fat or fat free)
1 cup of your favorite salsa

Meat filling:
1 lb. lean ground beef, ground turkey or vegetarian meat substitute,
1 Tbsp olive oil (optional)
1 small onion, finely chopped
2 cloves garlic, finely chopped
1 Tbsp Worcestershire sauce
2 Tbsp. chili powder
1 tsp. ground cumin

Cook meat until lightly browned, add remaining ingredients and cook until onions and garlic are tender, about 5 minutes longer. Allow to cool slightly, around 10 minutes.

To make the salad dressing, combine 1 cup sour cream with 1 cup salsa in the bottom of a large salad bowl. Mix well. Add chopped lettuce on top, followed by the beef mixture, cheese, green onions, black olives and tomatoes.

Toss salad immediately prior to serving. Add broken chips, if desired.

16. **Whole Grain Cheese Ravioli with Artichoke Hearts, Black Olives, & Pesto (serves 4)**
1 9oz container refrigerated whole wheat cheese ravioli
1 (5 – 7 oz) container prepared Pesto
2 Tbsp. sundried tomatoes, sliced
½ cup ripe olives, drained and halved
1 4oz can artichoke hearts, drained and halved
2 Tbsp. shredded or grated parmesan cheese
1 Tbsp. chopped fresh basil, optional

Cook pasta according to package directions. Drain. Add prepared pesto, sundried tomatoes, ripe olives, and artichoke hearts. Mix lightly to combine. Top with cheese and basil if desired.

17. **Super Simple Talapia (serves 4)**
4 talapia filets
1/3 cup Victoria Taylor's Toasted Sesame Ginger Seasoning®
2 Tbsp olive oil

Place the Sesame Ginger seasoning on a plate or pie pan. Press seasoning onto the tilapia filets. Cook filets in olive oil approximately 2 minutes per side, or until the fish flakes easily in center.

18. **Easy Red Beans & Brown Rice**
Uncle Ben's Converted Brown Rice
1 (16 ounce) package turkey kielbasa, cut diagonally into 1/4 inch slices
1 onion, chopped
1 green bell pepper, chopped
1 clove chopped garlic
2 (15 ounce) cans canned kidney beans, drained
1 (16 ounce) can whole peeled tomatoes, chopped
1/2 teaspoon dried oregano
Salt and pepper to taste
½ red onion, chopped
Pickapeppa® sauce

Cook rice according to package directions.

In a large skillet over low heat, cook sausage for 5 minutes. Stir in onion, green pepper and garlic; saute until tender. Pour in beans and tomatoes with juice. Season with oregano, salt and pepper. Simmer uncovered for 20 minutes. Serve over cooked brown rice. Top with fresh chopped red onions and Pickapeppa® sauce.

19. Turkey Burgers with Blue Cheese and Hot Sauce

1 pound lean ground turkey meat
1 Tbsp. olive oil
1 ½ tsp poultry seasoning
1 Tbsp. grilling seasoning, such as Pappy's 50% Less Salt
2 cloves fresh garlic, chopped or 1 tsp. chopped or minced garlic from a jar
3 green onions, finely chopped
1 stalk of celery with greens, finely chopped
2 Tbsp. spreadable butter
¼ cup hot sauce
1 cup reduced fat or nonfat sour cream, (I like Naturally Yours®)
½ cup blue cheese crumbles
Lettuce leaves
4 whole grain burger buns or sandwich rounds

Mix ingredients from turkey through celery. Form into 4 patties, each patty 1 inch thick. Heat a nonstick skillet over medium-high heat and cook burgers for 6 minutes on each side. Remove to a plate.

Wipe the pan clean and reduce the heat to low. Melt spreadable butter in the pan. Add hot sauce to the melted butter. Return the turkey patties to the skillet and flip to coat in the hot sauce-butter mixture. Place burgers on bottom of whole grain buns or whole wheat sandwich rounds.

In a small bowl, mix the sour cream with blue cheese crumbles. Top the burgers with lettuce and blue cheese sauce.

20. Artichoke, Tomato and Spinach Pizza (serves 4)

4 Tbsp. olive oil
3 cloves garlic, finely chopped

1 lb. refrigerated pizza dough (whole wheat preferably, such as Trader Joe's)
Salt and pepper
2 cups shredded mozzarella cheese (about 8 oz)
4 Tbsp grated or shredded parmesan cheese
One 13.75 oz can artichoke hearts, drained and quartered
1/2 pint grape or cherry tomatoes, halved
2 cups cleaned baby spinach, chopped (about 2 oz)

Preheat the oven to 450°F. Either grease a baking sheet or stone with oil or cover it with parchment paper.

Mix the olive oil and garlic. With oiled hands, stretch the pizza dough to fit the baking sheet. Spread 2 Tbsp of oil & garlic mixture on dough leaving a 1/2-inch border, then sprinkle with the mozzarella and 2 Tbsp of the parmesan.

Toss the artichokes, tomatoes and spinach with the remaining oil & garlic mixture and arrange on top of the cheese. Sprinkle the remaining 2 Tbsp. parmesan on top. Place the baking sheet in the oven and bake until the crust is crisp and golden, about 18 – 22 minutes.

21. <u>Fish Tacos with Mango Slaw (these are delicious)</u>
1 lb fresh or frozen orange rough, tilapia or other fish fillets
1 Olive Oil
1 Tbsp Butter (spreadable ok)
¼ tsp ground cumin or 1 tsp fresh cilantro
1 clove garlic

Make Mango Salsa and refrigerate until fish is ready to be served. Thaw fish, if frozen. Rinse fish and pat dry. Place fish in a single layer in a greased, shallow baking pan. Mix olive oil, butter, cumin or cilantro and garlic. Brush over fish. Bake in a 450°F. oven or grill and cook for 4 – 6 minutes or until fish flakes easily with a fork and internal temperature reaches 160°F. Remove from heat and serve with mango salsa and warmed stone-ground corn tortilla, or low carbohydrate or whole grain wheat tortillas.

Mango Salsa:
2 ripe mangos, peeled and diced into ½ inch pieces (if unable to find ripe mangos, may use canned peaches in juice, but not in heavy syrup),
1 medium tomato, seeded and diced into ½ inch pieces
1 green onion, finely sliced
2 cups finely sliced cabbage (can use prepackaged fresh sliced cabbage)
2 Tbsp. lime juice
1 tsp Agave nectar or 1 tsp natural cane sugar (optional)
1 jalapeno pepper (optional)
½ cup Ranch Dressing

Mix all ingredients, cover and refrigerate.

22. Simple Homemade Chili (serves 6)
1 lb. lean ground beef or ground turkey (may also use Soy-riso® or turkey sausage)
1 medium onion, chopped
Large can (28 oz) tomato sauce or puree
2 small cans tomato paste
2 Tbsp. chili powder
1 tsp. cumin
½ tsp. coriander
½ tsp. cayenne pepper
¼ cup Worcestershire sauce
2 15oz. cans kidney or pinto beans (reduced sodium if desired)
Salt and Pepper to taste
3 cups water

In large pan, cook meat. Add onion and cook approximately 5 minutes until tender. Add the rest of ingredients including the water. Heat to a slow boil, reduce heat to a simmer and cook at least 45 minutes, stirring occasionally.

23. Beef Stew (serves 6)
1 lb. lean beef (chuck, round) cut into 1" cubes
1 Tbsp oil
2 large potatoes, cut into 1-1/2" pieces

2 carrots, cut into 1" pieces
2 stalks celery, cut into 1" pieces
One small onion, chopped
1 can beef broth or 1-1/2 c. water
½ tsp. bottled brown bouquet sauce
1 bay leaf
For thickening: ½ cup cold water and 2 Tbsp flour
Salt and pepper to taste.

Cook and stir beef in oil in a 12-inch skillet or Dutch oven until beef is brown, about 15 minutes. Add 3 cups water, ½ tsp. salt and pepper. Heat to boiling; reduce heat. Cover and simmer until beef is almost tender, 2 to 2-1/2 hours.

Stir in potatoes, carrots, celery, onion, broth or 1-1/2 c. water, brown bouquet sauce and bay leaf. Cover and cook until vegetables are tender, about 30 minutes.

Shake the ½ cup cold water and 2 Tbsp flour in a tightly covered container; stir gradually into stew. Boil and stir one minute until thickened. Add salt and pepper to taste.

24. Crab Cakes
3 cups crab meat (fresh, frozen, canned or imitation Krab)
2 large eggs, beaten slightly
½ c. fine dry whole grain bread crumbs, plus 3 Tbsp. for coating
2 Tbsp. finely chopped green onions
1 Tbsp. parsley, dried (or 2 tsp. fresh)
½ tsp. celery salt
3 Tbsp. Mayonnaise
1 Tbsp. Dijon mustard

Thaw and drain crabmeat if frozen. Mix above ingredients except crabmeat, then mix in crabmeat. Shape into 8 patties.

Combine 3 Tbsp. stone ground corn meal with 3 Tbsp. whole wheat fine dry bread crumbs. Coat patties with cornmeal mixture. In a large skillet, heat 2 Tbsp. oil. Add crab cakes. Cook over medium heat about 3 minutes on each side or until golden and heated through. Add additional oil, if needed. Serve immediately with lemon wedge, cocktail sauce or tartar sauce.

25. <u>Roasted Sweet Potatoes (makes 4 servings)</u>
2 medium sweet potatoes, peeled and cut into 1 1/2-inch-thick rounds
1 tablespoon olive oil
2 large garlic cloves, minced
2 Tbsp fresh thyme leaves, plus 2 thyme sprigs for garnish (optional)
1/4 teaspoon salt
1/4 teaspoon red pepper flakes

Preheat oven to 450°F. In large mixing bowl, combine all ingredients and toss. Arrange potato slices in single layer on heavyweight rimmed baking sheet or in 13x9-inch baking dish. Place on top rack of oven and roast until tender and slightly browned, about 40 minutes. Serve warm or at room temperature, garnished with thyme sprigs.

26. <u>Chicken Stir Fry</u>
4 (4 ounce) boneless skinless chicken breast halves
3 tablespoons cornstarch
2 tablespoons soy sauce
1/2 teaspoon ground ginger
1/4 teaspoon garlic powder
3 tablespoons cooking oil, divided
2 cups broccoli florets
1 cup sliced celery (1/2 inch pieces)
1 cup thinly sliced carrots
1 small onion, cut into wedges
1 cup water
1 teaspoon chicken base or bouillon granules
Uncle Ben's Converted Brown Rice, made according to package directions

Cut chicken into 1/2-in. strips; place in a resealable plastic bag. Add cornstarch and toss to coat. Combine soy sauce, ginger and garlic powder; add to bag and shake well. Refrigerate for 30 minutes.

In a large skillet or wok, heat 2 tablespoons of oil; stir-fry chicken until no longer pink, about 3-5 minutes. Remove and keep warm. Add remaining oil; stir- fry broccoli, celery, carrots and onion for 4-5 minutes or until crisp-tender. Add water and bouillon. Return chicken to pan. Cook and stir until thickened and bubbly. Serve over rice.

27. **Fresh Berries with Sweetened Cream (makes one serving)**
Place 1 cup of fresh berries in a bowl. Top with ¼ cup light cream or half & half. Sprinkle with 1 tsp. Ideal® sweetenter.

28. **Sloppy Joes (serves 4)**
1 Tbsp. oil
1 medium onion, finely chopped
½ green pepper, seeded and finely chopped
1 stalk celery, finely chopped
2 cloves garlic, minced
Salt and Pepper to taste.
1 lb. ground beef, ground turkey or vegetarian meat substitute
1 can (15 oz) tomato sauce
¼ cup ketchup (low sugar, low salt variety if desired)
1 Tbsp. Worcestershire sauce
Whole grain buns or whole wheat sandwich "rounds"

In large skillet, heat the oil over medium-high heat. Add the onion, bell pepper, celery and garlic; season with salt and pepper. Cook, stirring frequently until the vegetables are softened, about 5 to 7 minutes.

Add ground meat or substitute. Cook, breaking up the meat with a wooden spoon until cooked through, about 6 to 8 minutes.

Stir in the tomato sauce, ketchup and Worcestershire sauce into the meat mixture. Simmer until thickened, stirring occasionally, about 6 – 8 minutes.

Spoon onto buns or sandwich "rounds". Serve immediately.

29. Chef Salad (Serves 4)
4 – 6 cups chopped lettuce
4 oz low fat cheddar cheese, cut into ¼" strips
4 oz low fat swiss cheese, into ¼" strips
4 oz lean ham (preferably without nitrates), into ¼" strips
4 oz roast turkey (preferably without nitrates), into ¼" strips
4 hard boiled eggs, peeled and cut in half
2 green onions, sliced
8 – 12 cherry or grape tomatoes (or diced whole tomato)

Dressing: Mix ½ cup Ranch Dressing with ½ cup milk. Place in bottom of large salad bowl. Add salt and pepper as needed.

Place lettuce in bowl and arrange the cheeses, meats, and eggs on top. Sprinkle with the green onions and tomatoes.

Mix immediately prior to serving.

Serve with Broiled Cheese Toasts on the side.

30. Broiled Cheese Toasts
Preheat broiler to 500°F.
8 – 12 whole grain Melba toasts
¼ - 1/3 cup grated or shredded parmesan cheese

Place toasts on a baking sheet. Top each with small amount of the parmesan cheese. Place toasts into broiler approximately 6 inches from heat. Broil for approximately 30 seconds to one minute, CHECKING FREQUENTLY TO AVOID OVERBROWNING.

31. Oven "Fried" Chicken
4 Chicken Quarters
3 cloves fresh garlic, minced or 1 Tbsp. pre-minced garlic from a jar
1 Tbsp. Olive oil
Salt & Pepper to taste
20 Whole Wheat Ritz crackers, crushed

Preheat oven to 375°F.

Rinse chicken, pat dry. Rub each chicken quarter with olive oil and garlic. Season with a small amount (1/4 tsp each) of salt and pepper. Coat each piece with cracker crumbs. Place skin side up on foil lined shallow pan. Bake for 35 - 40 minutes or until juices run clear when knife is inserted near the bone.

32. Mashed Red Potatoes
Pound red potatoes
Tbsp. spreadable butter or non-hydrogenated spread
2 – 4 Tbsp. milk

Cut potatoes into 1 inch cubes. Do not peel. Place potatoes in a pan of cold water. Add a small amount of salt. Bring potatoes to a boil and cook over medium heat for 20 – 25 minutes or until tender. Drain. Mash with a potato masher. Add butter and enough salt and pepper to taste. Gradually beat in enough milk to make light and fluffy.

33. Broiled Asparagus with Garlic
1 pound fresh asparagus
1 clove fresh garlic, minced or 1 tsp minced garlic from a jar
1 Tbsp. Olive oil

Preheat broiler to 450°F.

Break off the tough lower ends of the asparagus. Toss with olive oil and garlic. Add small amount of salt and pepper to taste. Arrange in a single layer on shallow pan and place in broiler. Cook for 5 – 6 minutes, carefully turning asparagus once.

34. Multilayer Mexicali Dip (serves 4 – 6)
One 15-1/2 oz can refried beans (or can use 2 cups homemade beans)
1 cup (8 oz) regular, low fat, or nonfat sour cream
1 cup salsa
1 cup reduced fat cheddar cheese
1 tomato, diced
1 avocado, cut into ½" cubes
1/2 cup sliced black olives

2 green onions, sliced
2 Tbsp. jalapeno peppers, diced (optional)

Spread beans onto a large plate or platter. Top with the remaining ingredients, in the order listed, ending with the optional jalapeno peppers. Serve with whole grain corn tortilla chips or bean chips.

35. <u>Smoked Salmon and Chive Omelet (Serves 2)</u>
4 eggs or 2 whole eggs plus 2 egg whites
1 Tbsp. finely chopped fresh chives or green onions
1 tsp. butter
2 oz smoked salmon, roughly chopped
Salt and Pepper

Break the eggs into a bowl and beat with a fork until just combined. Add chopped chives or green onions, season with salt and a generous sprinkling of pepper. Set aside.

Heat the butter in a medium nonstick frying pan until foamy. Pour in the egg mixture and cook over medium heat for 3-4 minutes, drawing the eggs from around the edge into the center of the pan from time to time.

At this stage, you can either leave the omelet slightly soft or you can finish cooking it under the broiler, depending on how you like your omelet. Top with the smoked salmon. Fold the omelet over, cut in half and serve.

36. <u>Spaghetti Carbonara (Serves 4)</u>
2 Tbsp. olive oil
1 small onion, finely chopped
1 large fresh garlic clove, crushed, or 1 tsp. crushed refrigerated garlic from a jar
8 slices pancetta or smoked bacon (preferably without sodium nitrates), cut into ½ inch pieces
12 oz dried pasta, such as Dreamfields®, Barilla Plus®, or whole wheat pasta
4 eggs or 1 whole egg plus 3 egg whites

6 – 8 Tbsp crème fraiche or Mexican table cream, heavy cream, or sour cream
4 Tbsp Parmesan cheese, plus extra to serve
Salt and Pepper

Heat oil in large pan, add the onion and garlic and fry gently for about 5 minutes or until softened. Add the pancetta or bacon to the pan and cook for 10 minutes, stirring often.

Meanwhile, cook the spaghetti in a large pan of lightly boiling water according to package directions, until just tender. Put the eggs, crème fraiche (or other cream), and grated Parmesan in a bowl. Stir in plenty of black pepper and beat well.

Drain the pasta thoroughly and gently add it to the pan with the pancetta or bacon and toss well to mix. Turn off the heat under the pan, then immediately add the egg mixture and toss thoroughly so that it cooks lightly and coats the pasta.

Season to tast with the salt and pepper and serve immediately with extra Parmesan cheese.

Chapter 10

Looking Forward to the Future

As consumers, how can we compete with these high-energy commercials and cute characters encouraging us and our children to eat these high in fat, high in sugar, and totally processed foods?

As for my own child, I talked to her often about the commercials and, from a very young age, tried to teach her about consumerism. I'd tell her, "You don't want to let these commercials try to control your brain and make you want to buy things, because that is what they are trying to do."

Now, at age eighteen, it does my heart good when we are walking past the doughnut aisle and she says to me, "It's funny, but I hardly even see those things any more."

As parents or just as health-conscious consumers, what can we do?

- ❑ Keep healthy snacks around the house (see chapter on healthy menus)
- ❑ Choose to dine out less often (aim for one time per week or less)
- ❑ Prepare family meals
- ❑ Limit the kid's TV, computer and video game (screen time) time (experts are recommending one to two hours per day)
- ❑ Teach yourself and your kids about consumerism, and learn how not to become a victim of advertisers

My business is not to remake myself. But to
make the absolute best of what God made.
—Robert Browning

Aggressive and Sophisticated Marketing of Foods by the Mass Media

The following image is from an advertisement from the USDA for the food pyramid:

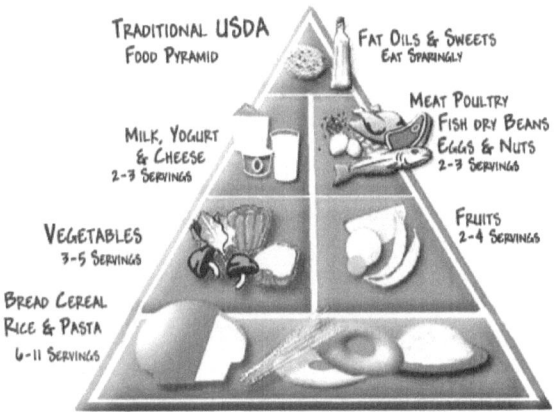

Traditional USDA Food Pyramid

Fat Oils & Sweets
Eat Sparingly

Meat Poultry
Fish Dry Beans
Eggs & Nuts
2-3 Servings

Milk, Yogurt & Cheese
2-3 Servings

Vegetables
3-5 Servings

Fruits
2-4 Servings

Bread Cereal Rice & Pasta
6-11 Servings

Now check out a sample image that may be used from the soft drink industry:

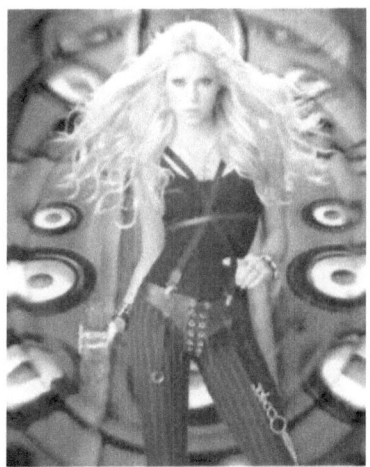

We've got to ask ourselves: Who is doing the best advertising?

In the documentary *Super Size Me* by Morgan Spurlock, the author presented preschoolers with pictures of various famous people and asked them to identify the people in these pictures. It was rather sad to see these children recognize pictures of Ronald McDonald more often than pictures of other famous faces, such as our current president, our first president, or even a picture of Jesus.

Kids are found to be quite influential in the purchasing habits of American families, and the findings is not lost on the advertisers. One study showed that a during a typical four-hour stint of Saturday morning cartoons, a child may see as many as 202 advertisements for junk foods. Other studies have shown that the more TV children watch, the more likely they are to snack between meals, eat foods shown on TV, and try to get their parents to buy unhealthy foods.

"This current generation may be the first in the history of mankind to live a shorter lifespan than their parents."

Source: *New York Time* article, 2005

As I said before, I believe the low carbohydrate diets almost had things right. Any diet that can get people to stop drinking 10-12 teaspoons of sugar in every twelve ounce soda cannot be all bad.

However, limiting foods that our God placed here on earth is not the answer. I have never, in 25 years of being a dietitian, seen anyone who could stick to the low carb diets long term.

> And God said, "Behold, I have given you every plant yielding seed that is on the face of the earth, and every tree with seed in its fruit. You shall have them for food."
>
> -Genesis 1:29 ESV

The problem of obesity is indeed multi-faceted, including our stressful lifestyles, our reduced activity levels, our increase in processed and fast foods, our increase in portion sizes, our obsession with thinness and dieting, and for many, the genetic predisposition for overweight (GPO).

However, while there is this genetic trait that causes some to gain weight faster than others, by following God's eating plan, learning to better handle our stress, making time to rest and to exercise (play), we can manage our GPO and not allow it to take our bodies into the level where we need to go on starvation diets or surgically alter our bodies in order to keep our weight at a reasonable level.

While lots of people are trying to blame our processed food industry on most of the nutrition woes of our country, I believe that much of this information is relatively new. Until recently, we really were not aware of the dramatic rise in our intake of added sugars and the deleterious effect these and other processed carbohydrates have on our health.

I believe that the food processing industry can play a big role in helping Americans improve their diets. I may be a dreamer, but I can visualize these influential companies working with our researchers and government organizations to show Americans how to be truly healthy. Admittedly, the almighty dollar influences many decisions of big business, but hopefully we can find some sort of balance. For the health of our society, we need to look less at the bottom line of making cheap, processed foods that have a tremendously long shelf-life.

Instead of attacking the food processing industry with lawsuits as happened with the tobacco companies, I believe instead in taking a more positive and proactive approach, working in conjunction with them to promote more natural foods.

I would love to see fewer white flours and processed sugars used in breads, breakfast, and snack items. It would be a truly wonderful thing if our food processing industry would work at making healthier foods taste really good. Simple things, such as using stone ground corn to make chips and tortillas would be a good start. I would like to see advertisements from these companies for healthier foods. Profits can be made with these less-processed foods, although perhaps at a lower level. The health and well-being of our country's future is at stake.

In the meantime, we as consumers can make the choice to not allow ourselves to become dependent on these cheap white flour and sugar products. We can work to find recipes that our families love that are healthy. We can grow some of our own fruits and vegetables or at least visit a local farmer's market and pick up some of this wonderful abundance that God has so graciously provided for us.

Bibliography

Alfenas, Rita C., and Richard D. Mattes. "Influence of Glycemic Index/ Load on Glycemic Response, Appetite, and Food Intake in Healthy Humans." *Diabetes Care* 28 (2005): 2123-2129. 30 June 2008

American Dietetic Association Daily Tips. "Glycemic Index: What is it?" (2004) 10 July, 2008. *http://www.eatright.org/cps/rde/xchg/ada/hs.xsl/ home_4456_ENU_HTML.htm*

Bikeyahdei' Yati', Dine. "Tribal Employee: Television Promotes Culture Loss." *Tribal Employee*. 17 Apr. 2008. 23 June 2008 <http://tribalemployee.blogspot.com/2008/04/effects-of-television.html>.

Borushek, Allan. 2007. Calorie Fat & Carbohydrate Counter. Costa Mesa, CA: Family Health Publications

Boyles, Salynn. "Nature Trumps Nurture in Child Obesity." *WebMD Medical News* (2008).

Callaway, C.W. 1990. The Callaway Diet. New York: Bantam Books

Chan, Ginie, and David L. Katz. *Diet in the Presvention and Control of Obesity, Insulin Resistance, and Type II Diabetes*. Diss. Amerian College of Preventive Medicine, 2002. 30 June 2008 <www.acpm. org/2002-057(F).htm>

Coulston, Ann M. "Cardiobascular Disease Risk in Women with Diabetes Needs Attention." *American Journal of Clinical Nutrition* 79 (2004): 931-932. 30 June 2008.

Cummings, Sue, Ellen S. Parham, and Gladys W. Strain. "Weight Management." *Journal of American Dietetic Association* 102 (2002): 1145-1155. 5 Aug. 2003.

"Does God Really Care What We Eat." *Crusador*. 10 July *2008 http://www.healthtruthrevealed.com/full-page.php?id=13014634112&&page=article*

"Fact Sheets: Rice." *Goodness Foods*. 16 June 2008 <http://dspace.dial/pipex.com/town/place/vu87/rice.shtml>.

Franz, Marion J. "Hot Topic: Glycemic Index" CDE of the Diabetes Care and Education dietetic practice group. American Dietetic Association (October 2005) *http://www.eatright.org/ada/files/GlycemicIndex.pdf*

Freeman, Janine. "The Glycemic Index Debate: Does the type of Carbohydrate really matter?" Diabetes Forecast. (September 2005) American Diabetes Association. *http://www.diabetes.org/glycemic-index.jsp*

Garnier, Lawrence, trans. "Do We Have to Ban Sugar?" Ifrance. 30 June 2008 <http://biorganic.ifrance.com/biorganic/sugar.htm>.

Hart, C.R., and Grossman M.K. 2001. The Insulin Resistance Diet. Illinois: Contemporary BooksIversen, Jeff. "White Bread." Aiming Higher. 30 Dec. 2007. 30 June 2008 <http://aiminghigher.blogspot.com/2007/12/short-history-of-white-bread.html>.

Kennedy, James J. 1999. "The Pima Paradox." 23 June 2008 <http://www.foodandhealth.com/cpecourses/giobesity.php#_Toc477841655>.

Krause, M.V. and Mahan, L.K. 1984. Food, Nutrition, and Diet Therapy. Philadelphia: W.B. Saunders CompanyPortion Distortion: Serving Sizes are Growing." *Meals Matter*. 23 June 2008 <http://www.mealsmatter.org/EatingForHealth/Topics/article.aspx?articleId=53>.

Last, Allen R. "Low-Carbohydrate Diets." *American Family Physician*. 16 June 2008 <http://findarticles.com/p/articles/mi_m3225/is_11_73/ai_n16546190/>.

Lasiter, Larry. "Food and the Bible" 10 July. 2008. Crusade Church of God *http://www.pointsoftruth.com/foodlaw.html*

Leach, Jeff D. "So Go the Pimas, So Go the Rest of Us." *Paleobiotics Lab.* 30 June 2008 <http://paleobioticslab.com/pima_diabetes.htm>.

Lichtenstein, A H. "Dietary Fat and Cardiovascular Disease Risk: Quantity or Quality?" *Journal of Women's Health* 12 (2003): 109-114. *PubMed.* 18 Aug. 2003.

"Macrobiotics: White Rice, White Bread." 30 June 2008 <http://macrobiotics.johreiki.net/blog-3232.php>.

Pettitt, D J., M R. Forman, R L. Hanson, W C. Knowler, and P H. Bennett. "Breastfeeding and Incidence of Non-Insulindependent Diabetes Mellitus in Pima Indians." *The Lancet* 350 (1997): 166-168.

Pietiläinen KH, Sysi-Aho M, Rissanen A, Seppänen-Laakso T, Yki-Järvinen H et al (2007) Acquired obesity is associated with changes in the serum lipidomic profile independent of genetic effects—a monozygotic twin study. PLoS ONE 2(2): e218. doi:10.1371/journal.pone.0000218

Schlosser, Eric. 2002. Fast Food Nation. New York: Houghton Mifflin

Sorensen, Thorkild I., and Soren M. Echwald. "Obesity Genes: Identifying Single Genes Involvedin Polygenic Inheritance is Not Easy." *British Journal of Medicine* (2001): 630-631.

Stunkard, A. J., T. T. Foch, and Z. Hrubec. "A Twin Study of Human Obesity." *Journal of the AmericanMedical Association* 256 (1986). 15 June 2008. Williams, Desmond E., and William C. Knowler. "The Effect of Indian or Anglo Dietary Preferences on the Incidence of Diabetes in Pima Indians." Diabetes Care 24 (2001): 811-816. 30 June 2008.

"Super Size Me." *Wikipedia.*

Veracity, Dani. "White Flour Contains Diabetes-Causing Contaminant Alloxan." *Natural News*. 2 June 2005. 30 June 2008 <http://www.naturalnews.com/008191.html>.

Visiol, F, and C Galli. "Biological Properties of Olive Oil Phytochemicals." *Critical Review of Food Science and Nutrition* 42 (2002): 209-221. *PubMed*. 18 Aug. 2003.

Willett, W C., F Sacks, A Trichopoulou, G Drescher, A Ferro-Luzzi, E Helsing, and D Trichopoulous. "Mediterranean Diet Pyramid: a Cultural Model for Healthy Eating." *American Journal of Clinical Nutrition* 61 (1995). 30 June 2008.

Winnail, Douglas S. "Bible Health Laws" *Tomorrow's World Magazine* 6 (2004) March-April

Zhang, Cuilin, Simin, Liu, Solomon, Caren, Hu, Frank. "Dietary Fiber Intake, Dietary Glycemic Load, and the Risk for Gestational Diabetes Mellitus." *Diabetes Care* 29 (2006): 2223-2230 American Diabetes Association. 10 July 2008.

Index

Stunkard, AJ, 44
sugar, 62, 72
  processed, 53, 98
sugar alcohols, 66, 72
Super Size Me, 95
sweeteners, artificial, 65
sweets, 70
syndrome X, 17, 48

T

taco, chicken, 76
tea, iced, 32, 35
toaster waffle, whole grain, 75
tomato, soup, 76
tortillas, 46, 71, 75, 77
Trail Mix, 75
turkey, 76
twins, studies on, 44

V

vegetables, 18, 22, 66–67, 75–77, 98
  fresh, 31–32

nonstarchy, 71
starchy, 54

W

water, 32
weight
  excess, 17, 34, 41
  gain, 30
  management, 40, 44
wheat, 22, 56, 75–77
Wheat Thins, 75–76
whole wheat, 56, 75, 77

Y

yogurt, light, 69–70